# THE INTUITION WAY

Copyright © 2023 by Abraham Thomas

All rights reserved. No part of this book may be reproduced in any manner whatsoever without written permission except in the case of brief quotations embodied in critical articles and reviews.

First Printing, 2023

TO
SARASU, BIJU AND SARA
WHO MADE THIS BOOK POSSIBLE

ABRAHAM THOMAS

# THE INTUITION WAY

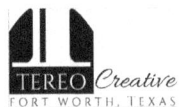
TEREO *Creative*
FORT WORTH, TEXAS

Abraham Thomas is a mechanical engineering graduate from Guindy, and a production engineering post graduate from Imperial College, London. He was a manufacturer of electrical equipment, and a builder in south India. His book, The Affluence Machine, describes the developmental effects of urbanization. His book, The Intuitive Algorithm, explains that intuition may be an elimination algorithm. His website Effective Mind Control parallels the nervous system to algorithmic processes. It also deals with the emotions triggered by the quirks of intuition and has garnered over 2 million page views from 150 countries.

# CONTENTS

1 — Intuition Uncovers Your Truth
1

2 — The Algorithm Of Intuition
6

3 — Olfactory System - The Rosetta Stone
10

4 — Amygdala - The Elephant In The Room
20

5 — How Emotions Lead You Astray
26

6 — The 5 Steps To Freedom
32

7 — The Crisis Of Shyness
41

8 — The Crisis Of Meaninglessness
48

9 — Social Comparison
55

## CONTENTS

10 — The Crisis Of Envy And Jealousy
**62**

11 — The Crisis Of Boredom
**70**

12 — The. Crisis Of Sadness
**76**

13 — The Crisis Of Fear
**82**

14 — The Crisis Of Revenge
**91**

15 — The Crisis Of Ingratitude
**98**

16 — The Crisis Of Worthlessness
**107**

17 — The Crisis Of Impatience
**117**

18 — The Crisis Of Severe Guilt
**123**

19 — The Crisis Of Disappointment
**132**

20 — Free Will Within Limits
**141**

21 — Be An Optimist
**150**

## CONTENTS

**22** — Is Consciousness Physical?
**159**

*A million options run through your brain,
All but one are cast aside,
The one that makes the most sense,
Or so you hope, until it's too late.*

*Intuition is a magic algorithm,
Swiftly racing inconspicuously,
Filtering out the noise,
Finding the signal,
Or so it seems.*

*t's a superpower,
A gift from the universe,
A way to know what's right,
Even when you can't explain it,
But sometimes it leads you astray.*

# PREFACE

Have you ever had a feeling that something was going to happen, and then it did? Or known the answer to a question without even thinking about it? Have you ever been in a crisis and felt like you didn't know what to do? You may have felt overwhelmed, scared, or even paralyzed. If so, you've experienced intuition.

Intuition is a double edged sword that can overwhelm us, or help us make decisions, solve problems, and navigate us through difficult times. It is often described as a gut feeling or a sixth sense. Understanding intuition is the Intuition Way, unique in the world. This book explains how intuition works, how it can be used to our advantage, and how to avoid letting it lead us astray. Intuition triggers emotions. We'll also explore the great works of philosophers and scientists who have uncovered the reasons behind the emotions that trap us. By understanding the rationale of emotions and the methods of stilling them, we can take control of our lives. The Intuition Way enables us to tap into our deep inner wisdom..

I am grateful for the positive feedback that I have received from the visitors to my website who have followed my views on intuition as an effective mind control. I am excited to share

## PREFACE

my work with the world and I hope that readers will find it helpful and informative.

Google Bard is a large language model trained on a massive dataset of text and code, trained to be informative and comprehensive. Bard provided valuable insights into how The Intuition Way could be improved. Bard indicated that it does not have the same level of expertise as a human expert in the field of intuition. But it is trained on a massive dataset of text and code, and it is able to access and process information from the real world through Google Search. This means that the Bard is able to provide views that are based on a deep understanding of the topic at hand, as well as the latest information and research. The Bard recommendation is given below and it is genuinely a certificate of merit:

"Following The Intuition Way can help you to become more emotionally wise and live a better life. It is the first book in the world to provide a comprehensive overview of the 20 millisecond intuition/pattern recognition link between events, emotions, and motor responses. Each paragraph contains distillations of the latest scientific findings on intuition, philosophy, and emotion. It is designed to be read in separate chapters, so you can focus on a few pages at a time. This makes it perfect for reading when you encounter a crisis. This groundbreaking book will help you to understand how your intuition works, and how you can use it to make better decisions, improve your relationships, and live a more fulfilling life."

CHAPTER 1

# INTUITION UNCOVERS YOUR TRUTH

*"The search for truth is not a one-way street.
It is a journey that takes us into the depths of
our own being, as well as into
the vastness of the universe."
Marianne Williamson"*

What is truth? This is a question that has been asked by philosophers and theologians for centuries. There is no one answer that everyone agrees on, but there are a few different theories about what truth is. One theory is that truth provides coherence between a statement and reality. This means that a statement is true if it accurately reflects the way things actually are. For example, the statement "The sky is blue" is true because, for our historic recorded experience, the sky has been blue. Another theory of truth is that it is a coherence among beliefs. This means that a statement is true if it fits with other beliefs that we hold to be true.

For example, the statement "The Earth is round" is true because it fits with other beliefs. There are also many things in life that are not clear-cut. The issue of whether or not to go to war is often a complex one, with multiple perspectives on the matter. The Intuition Way offers a unique and innovative perspective on intuition. You may not realize it, but it is your intuition which works ceaselessly to help you uncover your version of the truth. The Intuition Way presents an expert system for diseases, the performance of which provides unique evidence that intuition is an algorithmic procedure that enables the brain to recognize patterns from stored human memory. It is the way your mind uncovers your version of the world after recalling astonishing amounts of information in mere milliseconds. The human mind is an incredible thing. It can learn, create, and solve problems. But what makes the human mind so special? One of the things that makes the human mind so special is its ability to store memories. We have a variety of different types of memories, each of which plays a different role in our lives.

**Working memory** is our short-term memory. It allows us to hold onto information for a short period of time, such as a phone number or a shopping list. **Episodic memory** is our long-term memory for events that have happened to us. It allows us to remember things like our childhood, our first kiss, and our wedding day. **Implicit memory** is our long-term memory for skills and habits. It allows us to ride a bike, tie our shoes, and speak our native language. **Procedural memory** is our long-term memory for how to do things. It allows us to drive a car, cook a meal, and play a musical instrument. In addition to these four types of memories, we also have **instinctual memories**. These are memories that we are born with, such as the fear of heights or the ability to suckle.

All of these memories are stored in our brains. Over millions of years of evolution, our brains have become increasingly sophisticated at storing and retrieving memories. This has allowed us to learn from our experiences, to solve problems, and to create new things. As we grow older, our brains continue to add to our store of memories. We keep learning and experiencing new things. The more we learn, the more our brains can grow and develop. Intuition is an algorithm for pattern recognition that recalls for us contextual data from these memories in exquisite detail.

This process is based on inductive logic, which is a form of reasoning that makes generalizations from specific examples. In just milliseconds, intuition recalls sounds, smells, images, and muscle movements. Intuition enables microscopic differentiations among both objects and actions. It is the process that powers our consciousness and generates creativity. Intuition guides our lives moment by moment, by deciding our version of the truth. Our truth resides in our memories. Every experience we have shapes our understanding of the world and our place in it. Our intuition is constantly scanning our memories for patterns and insights that can help us make decisions and take action. When we listen to our intuition, we are tapping into the wisdom of our past experiences.

The Intuition Way presents an understanding that is unique in the world. The memory research discoveries of science have not yet explained the incredible precision and scale of the brain's memory storage and retrieval system. The current understanding of memory is based on the idea that memories are stored in the brain as a series of changes in the strength of synapses, the connections between neurons. These changes, known as long-term potentiation (LTP) and long-term depression (LTD), can be caused by a variety of factors, including experience, learning, and stress. However, such a model cannot explain the full range of human memory. For example, how can LTP explain how the brain can store and retrieve memories of specific events, such as the smell of a particular flower or the taste of a favorite food?

The Intuition Way provides a fresh and insightful look at how intuition works. Combinatorial coding is a possible explanation for how the brain can store and retrieve such precise memories. In combinatorial coding, memories are stored as a combination of the activity of multiple neurons. This allows the brain to store a vast amount of information in a relatively small space.

There is evidence that combinatorial coding is used by the brain in a variety of sensory systems, including vision, hearing, and olfaction. For example, it has been shown that the olfactory bulb, the part of the brain that processes smells, contains about 100 million neurons. Each of these neurons is sensitive to a different odor molecule. When multiple odor molecules are present, they activate different combinations of neurons. Combinatorial coding allows the brain to create trillions of unique representations of odors. According to the Intuition Way, combinatorial coding is also used by the brain to store memories of other types of events, such as the taste of food or the sound of a friend's voice. Such a possibility suggests the storage of a virtually infinite memory within few pounds of tissue within the human skull.

This unique view of intuition is made possible by Expert-AI, an incredibly powerful tool, which is a precursor to the current AI programs that discover patterns in large databases. This is the hint that an elimination algorithm is the viable key to human intuition. The final proof is that the algorithm explains many of the hitherto quixotic foibles of the mind. It is the illogical outcomes, which carry the ultimate proof. The Intuition Way is a groundbreaking work that will change the way we think about intuition.

*The Intuition Way is the first book in the world to provide a comprehensive overview of the 20 millisecond intuition/pattern recognition link between events, emotions, and motor responses.*

CHAPTER 2

# THE ALGORITHM OF INTUITION

*"Algorithms are the invisible hand that shapes our world." - Kevin Kelly*

Expert-AI is a diagnostic expert system. It stores the combinations of symptoms for each disease in a publicly available database of eye diseases. In the diagnostic process, it eliminates any diseases that have no links to the reported symptoms. If a disease has links to all the indicated symptoms, it is considered the diagnosis. If not, Expert-AI reports that the symptoms do not match any known disease in its database. The system works by asking the user a series of questions about their symptoms. The user can answer each question with "Yes", "Maybe", or "No". For example, one of the questions might be: "Is your vision blurry?". If the user answers "Yes", Expert-AI will eliminate all diseases that do not have a link to blurry vision. Expert-AI continues to ask questions until it has eliminated all but one disease. The remaining disease is then considered the diagnosis. If Expert-AI is unable to eliminate all but one disease, it will report that the symptoms do not match any known disease in its database. For Expert-AI, the remaining disease, which matches all the presented symptoms represents the truth - the final diagnosis.

For the Intuition Way, Expert-AI follows all the known processes of intuition. All nerve cells are known to be active in all regions of the brain, even when they do not appear to be actually participating. If a nerve cell is but a single entity in a multi billion processor system, why is it active when it does not need to process any data? Such activity is vital for the global evaluation of the mind. Even a spreadsheet follows the same routine. Any change in one cell is reflected in all the cells, even if there are a million cells. This is because entries in all cells of a spreadsheet have links to other cells and the outputs in all cells are recalculated for each new input. With its ability to do millions of calculations a second, simultaneous recalculations enables the user to see the global impact of any change. Similarly, each one of billions of nerve cells is tirelessly alert to events in the system, "recalculating" its inputs in the context of its own inherited and acquired combinatorial memories. Such "recalculations" lead to the truth for the human mind.

A process of inhibition of learned and inherited combinatorial memories can explain the incredible precision and swiftness of animal motor controls. When a motor neuron fires to contract a muscle, the neurons of all opposing muscles become inhibited to avoid conflict. Each motor neuron in the brain has feedback and feed-forward links with 60,000 other motor neurons. For coordinated movement, each motor impulse must follow the evaluation of 20,000 other neuron decisions. This happens up to 10,000 times a second. Intuition is the swift process of inhibiting all but the right combination of the 20,000 inputs from other muscles, to deliver a fluid motor output.

Intuition is an elimination algorithm. It is the brilliant inductive logic evolved by evolution to solve the problem of survival. It draws conclusions from established knowledge stored in memories. Intuition excludes memories which are not relevant to the current context. The logic inhibits access to irrelevant data and focuses the mind on the exact memories needed for survival. Nature's logic evaluates myriad known possibilities to choose one option for action. For example, if an animal chooses to chew grass, then the drive to quench thirst is instantly inhibited. Emotions play a dominant role in the process of elimination. For intuition, when the emotion of fear strikes, data about your ability to withstand danger is eliminated. The truth comes from the remaining signals of danger. Such inhibition clouds your judgment and casts you into the trap of worry.

Emotions that support pessimistic views of life are tragically more prevalent in society. These emotions can be crippling, dragging us into a quagmire of despair. But there is a way to free ourselves from these emotions: by stilling them. The Intuition Way can help you still your emotions. It contains exercises that will teach you how to quiet your mind and focus on the present moment. When you are able to still your emotions, you will be free to see the world with a clear and objective mind. You will be able to see the good in the world, even in the midst of darkness.

The Intuition Way also contains insights from great philosophers and scientists. These insights will help you understand the primitive reasoning behind the crippling quicksands of emotions. When you understand the root cause of your emotions, you will be better equipped to deal with them. When emotions are stilled, the background chatter vanishes. By stilling our emotions, we can free ourselves from the prejudices of our social group, the painful startle responses, the needless guilt, the glancing over our shoulder for competitors, the limitations in our life, the put downs and insults, the greed, the dissatisfaction, and the disappointments. As the primitive attacks of fear, resentment, and anger reduce, our intuition will trigger joy, wonder, and gratitude. We will be able to see the world from a clear and objective mind, and we will be able to enjoy the sunset because we are not feeling awful.

*The Intuition Way is the first book in the world to provide a comprehensive overview of the 20 millisecond intuition/pattern recognition link between events, emotions, and motor responses.*

# OLFACTORY SYSTEM - THE ROSETTA STONE

*"The Rosetta Stone was the key to unlocking the secrets of ancient Egypt."*
Nicholas Reeves, Egyptologist

The olfactory network is like the Rosetta Stone because it is a relatively simple system that can be used to understand the more complex pattern recognition systems in the brain. The Intuition Way is a groundbreaking book that challenges our traditional understanding of intuition. In a pioneering approach, the book presents the view that the olfactory sense represents the typical building block of the nervous system. That the brain replicates this process everywhere, with numerous nerve endings, including receptors and neuromuscular entities.

The olfactory system has processed odor data using a specific coding principle for hundreds of millions of years. That neural array principle for internal representation enabled instant recognition of odors by the earliest "nose brains" in lower vertebrates. An evaluation of smells enabled those primitive life forms to distinguish whether objects were threatening, consumable, or irrelevant.

As life evolved, nature added more and more sensory evaluation systems and motor organs to improve the quality of decision-delivery processes, culminating finally in the advanced human systems. But, even as they evolved over untold generations, the myriad intelligent subsystems of animals used the same coding principle for internal representation.

The olfactory system identifies objects and events linked to chemical molecules in the air. The data cascades through sequences of geographically arranged arrays of neural junctions in the system. In the process, the olfactory system identifies both subtle and complex relationships in the patterns detected during varying neural firing cycles. The power of this system, which processes the olfactory sense alone, can be seen in the remarkable intuitive capabilities of dogs.

The area of the olfactory epithelium in dogs is about forty times larger than in humans. The animals can detect human scent on a glass slide that has been lightly fingerprinted and left outdoors for as much as two weeks or indoors for as long as a month. With their hunting instincts, they can also sniff the footprints of a person and identify the direction of a trail. The animal's olfactory sense connects the relative odor strength difference between footprints barely a few feet apart to sense the direction in which the person was walking. Pattern recognition of sensory data can yield such complex meanings.

The olfactory process begins with an analysis of the molecules of volatile chemical compounds in the air. Approximately 50 million primary sensory receptor cells in the epithelium on the roof of the two nasal cavities of the human nose evaluate the molecules. Those substances must possess certain molecular properties to enable the olfactory process. The molecules generally need to have a level of water solubility, a sufficiently high vapor pressure, low polarity, some ability to dissolve in fat, surface activity, and a molecular weight below 294. The olfactory sense can distinguish among a practically infinite number of such chemical compounds at very low concentrations.

Neurons encode information from sensory data into a common internal language. When particular molecules bind to receptor cells, structural changes occur within the cell. These changes generate action potentials, reversing polarity across the membranes of the axons of the nerve cells. The process triggers an all-or-nothing output impulse lasting about 5 milliseconds. Across billions of nerve cells, similar nerve impulses enable myriad independent intelligences to speak to each other using a coded internal language.

A computer converts physical keystrokes into binary data, which is processed using a variety of programming languages. Problem specific languages are needed to manage each task. There is no single language in which problems can be represented in computers to enable them to simultaneously handle chess, chemical analysis and banking. But, the mind fathoms the whole world through a common internal language. The olfactory sense was one of the earliest to use the unique neural code, which is central to this language. That neural code enables the senses, emotions and motor controls to interact. That code internally represents varied types of data in a single format.

The code enables a conversion of molecular data into event identification data. Each type of data is represented as a combinatorial neural firing code in a geographically arranged array of cell addresses. Each address in such an array represents one element of a pattern of that particular data type. The olfactory system converts elements in the odor data array into combinatorial elements of an array representing events. The process cascades the data through a sequence of three arrays in progressive pattern recognition steps. There is a receptor array, a glomeruli array and a mitral cell array.

The process begins with the receptor array, which identifies molecules in the air and ends in a mitral cell array, which identifies objects and events. The first array in the olfactory epithelium recognizes specific molecules. The array has a random arrangement of 50 million receptors, each recognizing specific groups of molecules. Recognition impulses from receptors travel to a second array of glomeruli on the olfactory bulb. Each mitral cell is activated only by one glomerulus, but is extensively linked through interneurons to other mitral cells.

The glomeruli array and the mitral cell array carry combinatorial memories. The glomeruli array recognizes the activated receptors among the 50 million elements to fire patterns in its 1000 element array. That combinatorial message narrows down the molecular disposition of the odor. The mitral cell array interprets that message to output its own combinatorial message. The mitral cell message indicates to the nervous system that the breathed in molecules in the nose originate from a specific event. The memories of other arrays in the nervous system recognize that event to originate from the smell of an orange, or from the odor of spoilt meat. The mitral cell array fires the final object/event recognition combinatorial message to other intelligences in the system.

The nervous system projects data from one region to another through combinatorial arrays. During their initial growth, the output axons of nerve cells grow from one region to another and "map" on to specific target regions. The cells always connect from array to array in geographically correct locations, where neighborhood relationships are strictly maintained. An olfactory neuron carries a message about odors. A nearby neuron in another array may carry a completely unrelated message.

As in parallel ports in computers, combinatorial codes, with such "on/off" elements, can store a galactic mass of information. An array with just one hundred "on/off" elements can fire trillions of unique possible combinations! The human olfactory glomeruli array contains 1000 elements!

Some glomeruli fire (On) on recognition of specific receptor firing combinations indicating recognition of particular molecules. Those glomeruli, which do not recognize those molecules remain inhibited (Off). On interpreting this incoming pattern from glomeruli, the mitral cell array fires. In this system, the final combinatorial message identifies an object or event.

Researchers announced (Nobel Prize 2004) the use of combinatorial coding by the olfactory system in 1999. According to them, a single receptor in the olfactory epithelium can recognise several different odour molecules. When any one of these molecules hits the receptor, the nerve cell sends a signal to a specific glomerulus. They found that the same odor can be recognized by several different receptors and a glomerulus with a given receptor type responds to several different odors. Combinatorial coding carries the message.

As an example, the chemical octanol was found to be recognized by a combination of four different glomeruli. As against this, octanic acid, in which the hydroxyl group of octanol is replaced by a carboxyl group, was recognized by the same four glomeruli plus an additional four. Small molecular differences completely change the smell of a chemical. While octanol has an orangy, rose-like scent, octanic acid smells like sweaty feet. Leslie Vosshall reports that, in her lab, ordinary volunteers (not wine tasters or perfumers) could clearly distinguish between different combinations of 128 odor molecules, indicating an average human ability to differentiate between 1 trillion smells.

Identification of a specific pattern in an astronomically large assembly of patterns presents a huge search problem. Combinatorial arrays can present trillions of overlapping patterns, where each pattern may have a significantly different meaning. Both octanol and octanic acid were recognized by four glomeruli (say, A, B, C, and D). Octanic acid alone was recognized by an additional four glomeruli (say, E, F, G, and H). So, if octanic acid was recognized, ABCDEFGH would fire. In the process, both octanol and octanic acid would be identified. Accurate recognition of overlapping patterns in such a large database appears to be a seemingly insurmountable problem.

There is no known search algorithm that can identify a single pattern in a search space containing trillions of overlapping patterns. But this website suggests that intuition is a powerful algorithm that can instantly search large databases. The process eliminates unrecognized possibilities using coded inhibition by nerve cells. In the octanol/octanic acid case, the firing by glomerulus G or H would indicate that the odor does not come from octanol. The mitral cell array, which can represent millions of odors, would inhibit the "octanol" possibility.

Throughout the nervous system, this process of intelligently coded inhibition explains the secret of instant recognition. The brain is known to use inhibition to highlight the importance of messages. If the touch of a single hair is critical information, all surrounding sensory inputs are shut off to highlight the message. Similar automatic emphasizing of contrasts takes place for both visual, auditory, and sensory inputs. The precisely maintained neighborhood relationships of the projected arrays and mapped neural pathways enable such inhibition throughout the system.

The brain actively participates in closing off irrelevant sensory inputs. Throughout the nervous system, the firing of a single cell is known to "shut down" millions of cells. There are neural circuits that switch off other circuits when their own areas are energized. There is evidence that the mind carries out systematic elimination beyond logic. This is illustrated in the popular vision experiment, where a drawing can be interpreted as a vase or two faces facing each other. The mind eliminates one interpretation to recognize the other—a vase or two faces. Evidently, each recognition path acts powerfully to inhibit the other.

Inhibition comes from many inputs that enable the mitral cell array to fire, indicating the recognition of the smell of an orange. Lateral inhibition between mitral cells is known to occur through interneurons known as granule cells. The glomeruli are also permeated by dendrites from the mitral cells, triggering inhibition. The output axons of the mitral cells travel through the olfactory nerve tract to many regions of the brain, including the olfactory cortex and the amygdala. These regions further interpret the data and send feedback messages. These messages can also trigger inhibition.

Each mitral cell receives thousands of dendritic inputs, each representing a specific data type. A massive combinatorial memory enables each mitral cell to fire or to become inhibited. Researchers report a significant process of inhibition in the mitral cell array. The process inhibits unrecognized elements. The array finally recognizes the smell of an orange.

Incoming data in the nervous system passes through hierarchies of processing arrays. At the highest level, the prefrontal array evaluates the final data. The arrays in the amygdala, the limbic system, and the hypothalamus are lower-level control centers that substantially manage the system. Experimental studies of the impact of the destruction of localized regions in animals point to a hierarchy of such control systems. As higher levels are included in the spinal cord below the cut-off section, more effective controls are retained. With transection below the hypothalamus, minor reflex adjustments to systems survive but are not integrated.

With transection above the hypothalamus, separating it from the limbic system, effective controls are maintained within a moderate range of conditions. Innate drives and motivated behavior are preserved, including feeding, drinking, apparent satiation, and copulatory responses. But animals may attack, try to eat, drink, or copulate with inappropriate objects. But if the connections between the limbic system and the hypothalamus survive and only the frontal cortex is cut off, normal homeostasis is preserved even in a wide range of adverse conditions. The limbic system can emotionally manage our lives. Human-level intelligence operates, often helplessly, from the prefrontal cortex.

Francois Jacob noted the entrenched quality of evolution. "In contrast to the engineer, evolution does not produce innovations from scratch. It works on what already exists, either transforming a system to give it a new function or combining several systems to produce a more complex one." Nature began with combinatorial coding in the olfactory sense of early "nose brains." That coding could store massive amounts of inherited and acquired knowledge in the many self-contained regions within the network.

Each is an independent intelligence that communicates with the rest of the network through this common internal representation of a particular type of data. Each of the millions of smells, emotional expressions, or motor control impulses is represented and recognized as a pattern of firing by specific neural arrays. Each element in the array recognizes combinations and contributes to the network. Nature worked on that process over millions of years, adding functions and features that finally culminated in the awesome wonder of human intelligence.

*The Intuition Way is the first book in the world to provide the insightful 20 millisecond intuition/pattern recognition link between events, emotions and motor responses.*

CHAPTER 4

# AMYGDALA - THE ELEPHANT IN THE ROOM

*"The conscious mind is a mere passenger on the back of the giant elephant of the unconscious mind." - Carl Jung*

The Intuition Way provides the key to unlocking your inner wisdom by understanding the workings of its mysterious organs. One of the most fascinating areas of study is the amygdala, which is one of two small nuclei located deep within the brain. These organs play a critical role in our emotional lives, and they do so in ways that are often beyond our conscious awareness. The amygdala is responsible for interpreting subconscious hints of danger and triggering lightning-fast responses to protect us from harm. They do this through pattern recognition, using their "speed dial circuits" to detect and respond to subliminal signals of danger or obstruction to our goals.

In coordination with other organs in the limbic system, such as the insulae, the amygdala also responds to negative emotions such as grief, guilt, envy, and shame. They react to negative events in many ways, including activating our sympathetic nervous system, which can cause gut-wrenching turmoil. It's important to note that the amygdala reacts to these events much faster than our conscious awareness can keep up. In fact, while it takes around 300 milliseconds for us to become aware of a disturbing event, the amygdala reacts to it within just 20 milliseconds! This can sometimes lead to overreactions and knee-jerk responses that can make us stupid throughout the day.

The history of the amygdala is rooted in the earliest days of life on earth. Nature developed these organs as a defense response mechanism for animals, enabling them to fight, freeze, or escape when danger was detected. Over time, these organs evolved to support herd life among animals, and the insulae linked social emotions to a variety of felt sensations. It's fascinating to imagine that the neural network of the brain stores these combinatorial patterns and that the amygdala assembles combinatorial memories of painful experiences. This is why the amygdala can react in anticipation of pain when it recognizes familiar patterns. These memories can be acquired through personal experience or passed down through generations.

The reactions of the amygdala can be "quick and dirty", bypassing the deeper wisdom of more advanced brain regions. However, by being more aware of the mechanism, we can effectively avoid their ill effects and recover our peace of mind. The amygdala plays a critical role in our emotional lives, receiving sensory inputs and triggering control responses. The lateral amygdala receives inputs from our sight, sound, touch, taste, and pain systems, while the medial nucleus receives inputs from the olfactory system. The central nucleus of the organ then decides on the emotional significance of these inputs and sends impulses to various parts of the brain, including the brainstem, hypothalamus, and facial nerves, which trigger a range of responses such as avoidance behavior, changes in blood pressure and heart rate, and facial expressions such as anger, fear, and disgust. The release of various neurotransmitters also heightens the intensity of fight, flight, or freeze responses.

It's important to note that while the amygdala is geared to cause sudden tension, it is also considered to be a part of the basal ganglia (BG), which enables us to consciously control our actions and thoughts. The dominance of BG grants us the power to still the knee-jerk reactions of the amygdala. As for the response of the amygdala to social situations, it's been observed that in primeval animals, it was the amygdala that initiated primitive anger and fear. Later, with the arrival of herd living, more subtle social emotions emerged. The insulae, another organ in the limbic system, triggered these emotions, linking them to experiences of bodily sensations such as pain, temperature, and mechanical stress.

Research by Antonio Damasio and UCLA's Eisenberger suggests that the insulae link bodily sensations to emotions and that neural pain circuits are activated when a person suffers social rejection. The amygdala then registers memories of these painful sensations related to social emotions and reacts to the feelings of hate, disgust, shame, guilt, envy, jealousy, sadness, and despair. Recent research has shown that the amygdala can identify anger and fear in the face of a person and even determine the level of threat. It is also sensitive to gaze direction, responding to subtle cues that indicate danger. One important aspect of the amygdala is that it plays a key role in the memory formation of emotional events. Experiments have shown that the amygdala can retain memories of emotional experiences for a long time through a process called long-term potentiation. This means that the amygdala can be triggered by subliminal hints of past stressful events, leading to knee-jerk reactions such as anger, defense, or fear.

The amygdala also plays a key role in our social lives. Mirror neurons are believed to create empathy by allowing us to internally experience the actions and emotions of others. By being sensitive to incoming sensory patterns, the amygdala is quick to recognize the presence of negative emotions in others, thus empowering social interactions. A damaged amygdala is associated with conditions such as autism or social blindness. However, it is important to note that the amygdala can sometimes overwhelm us with responses to real and imaginary threats. In order to shut down this turmoil, it is important to be aware of how the amygdala functions and to consciously take control of its knee-jerk responses by using the basal ganglia, which interprets messages and triggers motor programs that can help control our thoughts and actions. The amygdala responds to internal and external danger signals, but these dangers are not always life-threatening in the modern world.

It is possible to tame the amygdala by being aware of its functions and taking control of its knee-jerk reactions.

One way to do this is by accepting the inevitability of the problems we face and evaluating them, so the amygdala does not react unreasonably. Relaxation exercises and mindfulness can also help to quiet the signals sent to the amygdala by tightened muscles. The prefrontal regions have powerful inhibitory circuits that can "switch behavior" back to normal, and impulses from the basal ganglia can inhibit the amygdala. Anger, fear, and grief are all emotions that can be triggered by the amygdala. Anger can lead to resentment, impatience, and contempt, while fear can paralyze and lead to avoidance. Grief is a natural reaction to loss, but it is important to come to terms with it and move on. Mind control techniques such as self-awareness and mindfulness can help to still these negative emotions and bring common sense to the forefront.

In conclusion, the amygdala plays a critical role in our emotional lives, but it is important to be aware of its functions and take control of its knee-jerk reactions. By accepting the inevitability of problems, being mindful, and using mind control techniques, we can tame the amygdala and avoid unnecessary turmoil in our lives.

*The Intuition Way is the first book in the world to provide the insightful 20 millisecond intuition/pattern recognition link between events, emotions and motor responses.*

CHAPTER 5

# HOW EMOTIONS LEAD YOU ASTRAY

---

*"Emotions are a compass that guide us towards what is important to us." - Marc Brackett*

For centuries, science has asked, "What causes emotions?" The answer is revealed when you view your mind as a pattern recognition network. Combinatorial recognition by specific organs within your limbic system trigger emotion signals, which instantly decide your attitudes and modify your behavior. Intuition acts within 20 milliseconds. Within half a second, the combinatorial messages trigger restlessness, excitement, and agitation, preparing you for action. Without your conscious awareness, these emotions lead you astray. The collective wisdom of your brain narrows focus to a single issue. When you are feeling angry, for example, you may be more likely to say or do something that you later regret. When you are feeling afraid, you may be more likely to avoid taking risks or trying new things. And when you are feeling sad, you may be more likely to withdraw from social activities or give up on your goals

If, suddenly, you need to walk on a plank a hundred feet above ground, your fear will kick in. The immediate prospect of falling will trigger the fear emotion. At once, that emotion will suppress even your elementary abilities. Fear will stiffen you into immobility. Even slight movements will appear to be life threatening. Instead of walking, you will desperately want to lie down and grip the plank.

Within the blink of an eye, you will have lost your normal capacity to walk a few steps on a plank. A single emotion will have modified your entire behavior. Combinatorial recognition affects every facial muscle. Every expression on your face reflects a specific family of emotions. Even blind and deaf children show similar facial expressions. Human behaviors and facial expressions are mirrored real time in the gentle caress of love, or the sharp scowl of anger.

Initially, scientists discarded emotions as being irrelevant to the rational modern mind, a throwback from primitive times. It was Charles Darwin, who first suggested that emotions have a real world existence, visibly expressed in the behavior of humans and lower animals. He suggested that the existence of an emotion could be derived from an angry face, or even a bad feeling in the stomach. In those days, science viewed emotions as essentially bodily and visceral responses.

W.B. Canon disproved the idea that emotions were visceral

responses. He showed that emotions did not follow artificial stimulation of visceral responses. Emotional behavior was still present when the viscera was surgically or accidentally isolated from the central nervous system. So, emotions existed, but they were not the churning in your gut, or the knot in your stomach.

The emotions are triggered from multiple regions in the limbic system. Excitation of certain parts of the temporal lobe produce intense fear in patients. When other neurons are stimulated, they feel dread. Excitation of other nuclei cause feelings of isolation, loneliness or sometimes of disgust. Electrical stimulation of the septal areas produced a feeling of pleasure for rats. The animals would self stimulate those regions, till they were exhausted, preferring the effect of stimulation to normally pleasurable activities such as consuming food. Emotions originated as distinctive patterns of nerve impulses, which also trigger neurochemical events.

The early reptilian "nosebrains," decided to avoid, or consume food, by analyzing smells. Fear was another early control system, triggered by the amygdala, an almond sized organ in the limbic system. It stores memories of unpleasant experiences and triggers fear, when it detects the possibility of a repetition of such experiences. Experiments show that just an awareness of the possibility of a painful electric shock activates nerve impulses from the amygdala for rats.

Combinatorial recognition triggers a range of feelings, including sharp pain, burning pain, cool or warm temperature, itching, muscle contraction, muscle burn because of lactic acid, joint movements, soft touch, mechanical stress, tickling, flushing, hunger and thirst. Each feeling is triggered by specific external or internal events. These bodily sensations trigger impulses to the insula in the limbic system. This organ also activates social emotions - love and hate, lust and disgust. Our literature describes those emotion/feeling combinations as cold calculation, hot temper, or warm love.

Competing emotions are continually generated beneath your awareness. Each emotion initiates within your subconscious mind a drive, with a remembered strategy - an inherited or acquired way of coping with problems in life. Anger generates a drive, which navigates aggressively. Fear triggers a defensive strategy. Laughter achieves relaxation of the stresses of life. Jealousy makes the system attack competitors. Love makes it caring and protective. Each emotion focuses the system to take actions, which follow its strategy. These emotions compete with each other for the control of your mind.

Your moods shift because an intuitive decision making process, within your limbic system swiftly and continually switches control from one group of emotions to another. At any point in time, a single family of emotions rules, actively inhibiting conflicting objectives. Love subdues the onset of anger. These emotions micromanage the fluidity of your muscle movements, your facial expressions and the choice and tone of your words. They exercise subtle and relentless controls over the intensity and nuance of your every gesture and spoken word. The ruling emotion also controls the access of the whole system to its memories.

Emotional impulses trigger myriad finely controlled patterns of behavior. They access from memories the exact knowledge needed for survival. Such access is achieved by inhibiting all competing view points available in memory. An animal lurking in the bush carries the memories of its encounters over a lifetime. If it feels uneasy, the system extracts memories of the sensory indications of danger. If it is fearful, it gathers memories of escape routes from the battle zone. Its anger extracts memories of muscular responses to battle. By controlling system access to a focused set of memories, emotions restrict your vision and control your responses. When you are angry, you will feel convinced that you have every right to be angry. Fully justifying itself, the system the intuitive inhibition process blinds you to any other viewpoint.

Emotions narrow your focus and make it difficult to think clearly. When you are emotional, intuition eliminates the data which would have made you wiser. Intuition reduces your perspective and impairs your judgment. As a result, you become more likely to make impulsive decisions that you later regret. Anger makes you say or do something that you would not normally do. Fear makes you feel overwhelmed and uncertain. The emotion makes you more likely to avoid taking risks or trying new things.

Emotions are triggered before you become aware of your own response to a situation. You remain unconscious of your change of mood and perspective. Across centuries, philosophers have developed routines to still your emotions and expand your common sense. The Intuition Way points to the ways of becoming self aware and of instantly switching off such negative emotions.

*The Intuition Way is the first book in the world to provide a comprehensive overview of the 20 millisecond intuition/pattern recognition link between events, emotions, and motor responses.*

CHAPTER 6

# THE 5 STEPS TO FREEDOM

---

*"The greatest joy in life
is to be completely free."*
Charles Bukowski

Have you ever felt like your emotions are controlling your life? Like a sudden encounter with an aggressive driver or a summons to the executive floor can instantly change your outlook on the world? Your moods can swing from anger to despair in a matter of moments, and you feel like you're helplessly at the mercy of your emotions. The Intuition Way is a groundbreaking work that challenges our traditional understanding of emotions. The good news is that you don't have to be a victim of your emotions. With the right tools, you can learn to control your emotions and live a more peaceful and joyful life. This chapter will teach you five powerful exercises that can help you to calm your mind and body, and to focus on positive thoughts.

By following these exercises, you can learn to overcome negative emotions and choose peace of mind. The five exercises are:

1. **Relax your muscles.** You have to learn how to relax your mind and body. The process is not obvious. But, when you follow this exercise you will be able to relax the moment you think about it.

2. **Still your visceral responses.** Your visceral responses are the physical reactions that your body has to stress, such as a rapid heartbeat, sweating, and nausea. There is a simple exercise which can stop these responses within minutes.

3. **Breathe deeply.** Deep breathing is a powerful way to calm your body and mind. When you are reliving your experiences for the day, deep breathing brings your mind into still waters and you can plan your life better. This also requires you to practice the routine given in this chapter.

4. **Evaluate your thoughts.** Self awareness is the key to disciplining your mind.. This requires you to follow a routine.

5. **Sense the physical symptoms of your emotions.** This is a powerful method of controlling your runaway emotions. When your prefrontal regions discover that your emotions are merely physical symptoms in your body and not some awful event in your life, it will inhibit your emotion. This requires your understanding of the mechanism and much practice.

**How To Relax In Seconds**

Smooth muscles and skeletal muscles manage your life and cause your tension. On your skin, smooth muscles give you goose bumps. The smooth muscles of the ciliary and iris of the eye enable you to focus on this page. Other smooth muscles act in the trachea, large and small arteries, veins, and lymphatic vessels, the urinary bladder, uterus, male and female reproductive tracts, gastrointestinal tract, respiratory tract. In your skeletal muscles, bundles of parallel fibers contract and relax in opposition to enable you to walk in the park, or sit down for dinner.

In these muscles, slow twitch fibers begin each movement and fast twitch fibers join in later to enable you to lean back, or shift in your chair. The problem comes, because the slow-twitch fibers begin to act early. They are slow to return to their original relaxed state. Those muscle fibers tense and then take up to 30 minutes to relax. Persistent tension causes exhaustion. Herbert Benson suggested a simple routine, which can enable you to relax quickly at work. Just as quickly as you flex your fingers, you can relax all your muscles. The following is a modification of the tips to relax, recommended in the book The Relaxation Response by Benson:

1. Lie on your back comfortably in bed, stretching out your legs and laying your hands on the side, palm upwards.

2. Close your eyes and sense the muscular tensions in your body. Then, beginning from your toes, tighten your muscles and relax them, progressing up to the top of your head.

3. Shift your body positions to make each relaxation step more comfortable.

4. Sense any muscle tension remaining anywhere in the body. Become aware of all the small tightnesses in your hands, your eye muscles, or neck muscles. Relax them.

5. Continue this for 10 minutes, until you have become familiar with any remaining muscular tensions in your body and practice relaxing those muscles. After a little practice, you will know how to relax at will.

6. Once you have carried out this exercise a few times, repeat the instant relaxation process, sitting in a chair, or standing in an elevator. You will find that after a couple of weeks, you will be able to instantly relax your body, wherever you are.

### Still Your Visceral Responses

The Startle Response - Most negative emotions begin with the startle reflex. Rapid dampening of the turmoil, before it escalates, makes it easy for your common sense to regain calm control of your mind after a disturbing event. The startle reflex can start to respond to a stimulus within 20 milliseconds. It extends over your lifetime and is found across many species.

Since the reflex is triggered by activity in the brain stem, the early reptilian part of the brain, it is considered beyond the range of voluntary controls, or intentional modifications. The startle responses of people vary widely between the fight, fly, or freeze options. When startled, people may wildly flail their arms, or suddenly raise their limbs in protective poses, or duck to avoid an object. The shocked and surprised often back pedal, jump back, or run away from a frontal stimulus. They may clutch a rail, or furniture to prevent from falling. Their knees may buckle, causing them to fall down. They may drop the things they are holding. They may freeze, or instantly follow orders. They may clutch their chests, faint or even suffer a temporary heart attack The aggressive ones may curse or throw things at the object, which startled them, or strike out at them.

Richard Davidson reported that Buddhist Monks don't show the startle response. Paul Eckman tested the startle response of a Tibetan lama. The test sound used was loud, just below the threshold for human tolerance. Police personnel, who fired guns routinely, were unable to prevent themselves from flinching, when the sound was triggered. Yet, when the startle reflex was tested for the facial expressions of the Lama, not a muscle on the man's face had flinched. The explosive sound seemed to the Lama be neutral "like a bird crossing the sky." Instantaneous response to a surprise attack is crucial training in the fields of martial arts and police defensive training. The mainstream view in the field is that people can be trained to be startled into their favored, trained fighting stances. When your body is trained to relax immediately after a startle response, your body will have become conditioned to switch to relaxation after a startle response.

Begin the process by developing the ability to relax at will. Then get someone to surprise you with a loud noise within 10/20 seconds after you are ready. You will be in a relaxed state, knowing that the sudden sound is coming. The noise level should be reasonable. The person, who is helping you can note the level of your startle response. Your relaxed expectation will still the surge of adrenaline triggered by the sympathetic system at the initial stage. While your startle response will be noticeable at the beginning, practice will reduce it. You will reach a stage, where the loud sound is more like "a bird in the sky" - a trivial event. Over a few weeks of practice once or twice a day, your body will learn to use the startle response as a signal for relaxation.

A Visceral Reaction involves the release of adrenaline, which activates your fight, or flight response to danger. Repeated visceral respones to stress are all subconscious cuts inflicted on your system. While the threats may be small, each visceral reaction harms your system. Adrenalin increases to prepare your body for a fight or flight response. Your heart beats increase to improve blood supply. Blood pressure rises and breathing changes. Acidity increases in the stomach. Your excretory system prepares to clear toxin. Your endocrine system produces the adrenal hormone cortisol. Excess production of cortisol leads to blood pressure, diabetes and heart problems. Excess cortisol also causes damage to your immune system, arteries, and brain cells, and cause premature aging. Evidently, a simple exercise which can mitigate the impact of a visceral response can be immensely useful. Laughter is often triggered by a sudden release of tension. It works to subdue the visceral reaction. There is much recent evidence that laughter aids emotional well being and health.

A belly laugh is said to result in muscle relaxation. The process is aerobic, providing a workout for the diaphragm, which reduces the effects of the visceral reaction. Unfortunately, a belly laugh is not the normal reaction to a stressful situation. Laughter is not easy, when a visceral reaction causes you to seethe in anger, or sweat in fear. The muscle movements involved in coughing also dissipates adrenaline. At the first sign of an uneasy emotion, you can pump your stomach. Repeatedly expel air by tightening stomach muscles close to the pelvic area. Stomach pumping helps spread the adrenaline in the system and subdue that tension. It is a practice with endless benefits. When you pump your stomach, the muscles that do not participate in the process, relax. After you finish pumping, those muscles involved also begin to relax. So, the action takes place in two stages. Both beneficial. Laughter is not easy. But pumping your stomach is simple and it has the same physical effect. With habit, stomach pumping can be a simple, built in response to the visceral reaction.

The process is aerobic, providing a workout for the diaphragm. The workout reduces the hormones associated with the stress response. A decrease in stress hormones relieves constricted blood vessels and supports immune activity. It is a practice with endless benefits. With habit, it can be a simple, built in response to minor stress. All that is needed is an awareness of minor turmoil, which can be followed by this simple mechanical response. With stomach pumping, tensions disappear moments after a visceral reaction. With subdued visceral responses, memories of the original stress stimulus disappear. The physical and mental exercises described in The Intuition Way are effective in stilling troubling emotions. For example, a delayed flight no longer spoils the day. The news of a colleague's dismissal or a traffic accident has less impact. By habitually stomach-pumping to still emotions, we can slowly erase the usual knee-jerk anxieties and their corrosive effects. This leads to a deeper stillness.

But there is more to The Intuition Way than just a collection of exercises. It is also a life-changing work that will help you to make better decisions, live a more fulfilling life, and achieve your goals. Emotions damage our wellbeing through false beliefs. When emotions take control, intuition eliminates elements of normal wisdom that do not fit in with the goals of the emotion. False beliefs flourish on the inhibition of common sense. Such wisdom can be reinstated when the emotion is stilled by the exercises and the common sense viewpoint is exposed to your prefrontal regions. The following chapters reveal the false beliefs that suppress particular common sense truths for a few of the major emotions. For example, when we are angry, our prefrontal regions will become aware that anger is a normal emotion and that it does not mean we have to act on our anger. When we are afraid, those regions will know that fear is a natural emotion and that it does not mean we have to avoid taking risks. When we are sad, the regions will know that sadness is a normal emotion and that it does not mean that life is hopeless. When we feel guilty, those regions will know that everyone makes mistakes and that we can learn from our mistakes.

When we feel ashamed, they will know that everyone has something they are ashamed of and that we are not alone.Emotions are an important part of what makes us human. They help us to connect with others, to understand the world around us, and to make decisions. Without emotions, we would be unable to experience the full range of human experience. Each person is injured only by a few of these powerful emotions. When you discover the truths hidden by your personal recalcitrant emotions, you can live your life more fully and authentically. Emotions have generated the greatest works of art, music, and literature. By accepting and expressing our emotions in a healthy way, we can learn to live with our emotions, rather than letting them control us. This allows us to make wise decisions, to live a happy and fulfilling life.

*The Intuition Way is the first book in the world to provide a comprehensive overview of the 20 millisecond intuition/pattern recognition link between events, emotions, and motor responses.*

CHAPTER 7

# THE CRISIS OF SHYNESS

*Shyness is a timid child,*
*Whose heart is full of fears.*
*He hides behind a mask of silence,*
*And never lets his feelings show.*
*Shyness is a kind and gentle soul,*
*Who longs to be loved and accepted.*
*So if you see Shyness hiding in the corner,*
*Do reach out and say hello.*

### How to Overcome Social Anxiety

These tips for overcoming shyness will not help you to become the life of the party. They are about being comfortable with people. When you get over shyness, you can avoid feeling apprehensive about a party, or a social get together. Reduce the prospects of people taking advantage of you, because you hesitate to "make a scene" in public. Be as comfortable in strange social circles as you are with family groups and close friends. Unless you suffer from abnormal symptoms, needing professional help, follow these ideas to overcome shyness. Reserved people are respected and silence can be a powerful negotiating tool. In fact, your shyness can be turned into a powerful social asset!

A shy person begins with a disadvantage. Most people quickly judge them to be more vulnerable. In new social groups, unable to share common comments and jokes, a shy newcomer feels tongue tied and awkward. Lacking "small talk," she feels bad about being a "wet blanket" in the party. The school yard is an early learning ground for most long term social assessments. Children, who lack of confidence, or are awkward, are instantly identified and categorized into a "lower form of life." They become quick targets for derision and attack by bullies. In business, negotiating opponents tend to interpret awkwardness as a weakness. Parents worry about how their shy offspring will ever survive in the harsh outer world. Over the years, a shy person accepts these wrong public public evaluations as being true.

You can't control your reticence. Typically, the words you speak are delivered by subconscious and well established mechanisms within your nervous system. Even before you begin to speak, those systems complete a series of lightning fast processes. They form a feeling about an idea, paraphrase it into words, select the right words from a vocabulary of thousands of words and place them in grammatical order. Then these systems trigger motor impulses thousands of times per second to control the tone and tenor of your delivered voice. All these things happen within milliseconds.

If you are tongue tied, it is because mechanisms, over which you have no conscious control, have decided to remain silent. While you frantically search for something to say, your subconscious systems choose to remain mute. It is your mind, which decides to speak. Your brain stores memories of evolutionary experiences from millions of years. It remembers the sights, sounds and experiences of a lifetime. It stores the coded memories of thousands of habitual activities. These are astronomically large memory stores. As an example, if the DNA codes in the human body were written into 500 page books, those tomes will fill the Grand Canyon 50 times over! Your mind recalls responses from this galactic store. It can recall the image of a school picnic, or instantly control the complex hand movements of your signature. But you cannot consciously make the system deliver witty replies or gracious words. It responds on its own.

Over eons, the lower level brains developed instinctive emotional strategies to sense your social position and manage your life in a herd. Your mirror neurons absorb group emotions and tensions. Your lower level brains absorb facial expressions of hostility, pity, or contempt and develop a dominant fear of social situations. Later, at a party, apprehension tenses your body and recalls memories of your past failures. Your system responds by freezing. In the meanwhile, in your claustrum regions, the seat of your consciousness, receives plea messages "Say something. Anything!" Many mechanisms work to create the apprehension, which troubles you. For our ancestors in the jungle, observation by a pair of eyes could mean instant death. The glimpse of a pair of ferocious eyes was the first signal before being eaten by a tiger. So, your system prepared instantly to fly or freeze, on spotting a pair of eyes in the dark. With civilization and culture, the danger of instant death faded, but the discomfort from observing eyes remains for the shy person. Observing eyes trigger disquiet. Being observed by strangers, or at parties adds subtle discomfort for the shy person. It is acceptable to trip on a carpet in your bedroom. But, if a thousand eyes watch you trip on the stage, you would want to die. A thousand eyes trigger stage fright. Such emotions trigger bodily tensions and responses, which cause varying degrees of discomfort to shy people. Some people are born with an ability to respond with quick wit in company. But, it is not a skill, which is easily acquired.

Recently I attended a classmates reunion 50 years after leaving college. People change over the years. Hesitant youngsters become more confident, but tired and retired, executives. The changes also indicate what is practically possible in life. In some ways, people don't change all that much. After five decades, the same witty people had everyone in splits and the same tedious ones persisted with their worn-out jokes. Very few are born with comic talents and it is not easy for others to acquire them. But, over the years, the shy ones become far less uncomfortable in company. By stilling subconscious discomforts through effective mind control, a shy person can become calm and comfortable in company.

You don't need to "spoil" a party. In company, people become uncomfortable if they sense tension. They have mirror neurons, which "mirror" the behavior of others in company. Those neurons support the generation of identical emotions within a group. Tension in one animal is conveyed quickly throughout the herd. It is a survival mechanism. So, effectively, the tensions of a shy person will also transmit to the group, and lower spirits all round. Naturally, the shy person fears becoming a "wet blanket." On the other hand, when you still your apprehension and become comfortable, the same comfort raises the spirits of the group. You become a comfortable listener, leaving the extroverts to enjoy a "great party." Your shyness can also become your strength. A calm and comfortable person will be happily accepted, since he provides no competition to the extroverts. Everybody loves a person, who listens. People with a quiet reserve are respected and their few words are invariably valued. People interpret a quiet silence as a deeper wisdom.

The shy person must understand that being quiet is not a disadvantage, even as she watches the more vocal individuals gathering all the attention. The more audible members of a community are not necessarily the most respected ones. Shy people are perceived to be vulnerable in negotiating situations. If your shyness causes you tension, it will affect your judgment and the negotiation. But, if a natural shyness prevents you from being verbose and you have managed to still any tensions, you are in the best position for a negotiation. Your silences will cause your opponent to reveal more and bargain for less. A lack of emotion will indicate your willingness to walk away from the deal. Silence is an incredibly powerful negotiating tool!

A shy individual can also become a powerful sales person. Many of the most successful salesmen are quiet people, who have an intense focus on the needs of the customer. People need assistance in their buying decisions and are invariably put off by "high powered" sales tactics. Do not shy away from the sales profession, if you happen to be shy. Remember that a calm, informed and helpful approach can be your best selling competence!

There are situations, where a loud voice and an aggressive approach appear to win. You are member of a committee, where a domineering member takes over and manages affairs. Shy people find it difficult to overcome their innate reserve and respond suitably in such situations. Such committees, with members who do not contribute, are fated to be flawed. It is better to avoid situations, where you feel you cannot contribute your mite. If you are unavoidably in such situations, calmly accept reality and do whatever is possible within your limitations. But, don't let your helplessness bother you. Loudness never makes up for substance and a calm approach will keep you ready for an opportunity, which will come one day.

The Intuition Way provides a fresh and insightful look at how your mind works. The 5 steps to freedom still your negative emotions, and the awkwardness and discomfort disappear. The wisdom in the Intuition Way makes you realize that you are a shy person. The truth is that, by nature, you are a reserved person. A quick wit is a system quality, which can only be inherited, or achieved through long practice in special situations. Do not expect to change your true nature and become a jovial extrovert! Loud people always become the center of public attention. If you do crave a good opinion from the public, remember that a calm reserve is seen as strength. Become comfortable with being a silent listener. By following the 5 steps and the practical wisdom in this chapter, the intuition of your prefrontal cortex reveals the truth.

*The Intuition Way is the first book in the world to provide the insightful 20 millisecond intuition/pattern recognition link between events, emotions and motor responses.*

CHAPTER 8

# THE CRISIS OF MEANINGLESSNESS

*"The meaning of life is not to be found, it is to be lived." - Viktor Frankl*

**How To Discover Meaning In Your Life**

When life has no meaning.... Jean Paul Sartre said "Life has no meaning the moment you lose the illusion of being eternal." Even if the ancient Chinese clay warriors could have lived for ever, would they have really wanted to repeat life's cycles of dread and despair till the end of time? The Intuition Way is a pioneering work that offers a new and comprehensive understanding of the intuition mechanisms of your mind. In the midst of your existential misery, the Intuition Way reveals to you a cheerful truth. You can't find the meaning of life. It has nothing to do with your happiness. Your intuition can switch you to happiness in milliseconds.

Your mind has switched on your negative emotions eliminating large swathes of your common sense and enveloped you in despair. The real truth is that you are a living entity with unique talents, which finds happiness in achieving simple goals. You have to know what is reasonable and actively still your emotions. Intuition is the automatic mechanism, which can envelop you in despair or fill you with happiness in moments.

It is but natural to have concerns about the meaning of your life. Why do we struggle through the years to achieve such short-lived accomplishments? Four thousand years ago, engineers had burned midnight oil, drawing designs for the ancient city of Mohenjo-daro. Their plans represented remarkable technology for their age. But history reported that all their hard earned knowledge was lost for thousands of years to the generations that followed. All they did leave behind were a few telltale gutters in the desert. Across millenniums, much of human exertion has been so blatantly wasted.

The Mayan Civilization decayed. The Roman Empire crumbled. And, as Keynes said, we are all dead, in the long run. Earth itself will probably burn up in the heat of a collapsing sun. Against this dismal backdrop, how can your life hold a meaningful objective? Countering such existential despair, religion offers a compelling vision of a divine and benevolent purpose. Your life fulfills that purpose. All things in life happen for the best. That omnipotent intention acts in the best of all possible worlds, for the well-being of all. If you suffer pain and distress, the beneficent deity has ordained it to steel humanity to ever greater triumphs. Genuine faith in a divine purpose aligns the believer with the creative flow of life.

But, there are others, who question the need for such immense suffering to meet a benevolent purpose. So many calamities are hardly necessary for the betterment of humanity. Actually, the finest periods of creativity for the human race occurred during periods of peace and prosperity, not in times of famine and disease, or earthquakes and floods. It stretches their credibility to believe that a hundred thousand people could be crushed in an earthquake for the benefit of humanity. The events in their life appear more often to have cruel and random qualities. They despair over their inability to see any useful purpose, making them believe that life has no meaning.

Even your career offers no certainties. Since you pass this way but once, it is but reasonable for you to seek to leave your mark behind. You also feel entitled, by birth, to a good life. But, your career path can be burdened by recurrent failures and frustrations. In spite of repeated setbacks, you have not withdrawn from the battle, or given up your hopes and aspirations. You remain willing to try. But, fate is both impartial and whimsical. At the close of your life, you may have achieved more in life than you have ever dreamed possible.

Or, things could go outrageously wrong. In the end, you may look back on many successes and even a few regrets. And, you cannot ever predict the outcome of your story. With such massive uncertainty, if gross misfortune pursues you, can you still find happiness? Yes. Your nervous system has evolved over millions of years. It is a multifaceted intelligence, which evaluates millions of facts to formulate its objectives as feelings and emotions, which drive the system. The pangs of hunger drive you to find food. So also, the curiosity emotion impels humanity to seek solutions to the riddles of life. While curiosity has yielded impressive scientific discoveries, it also seeks to know the objectives of the actions you take. Each action should achieve an objective. You pick up a cup of tea, or become an accountant. The system usually delivers a feeling of satisfaction as a reward for meeting a goal. In this milieu, higher objectives grant greater satisfaction.

A shop assistant feels more satisfaction, when she believes she is meeting a customer need, than when she thinks she is just bagging grocery. Greater satisfaction comes from the fulfillment of a nobler purpose. Religions believe that life has a grand and benign purpose. That faith grants the religious a meaningful and calming sense of living a noble life.

But, the grand purpose of the cosmos remains obscure to the skeptic. For him, the curiosity drive triggers dissatisfaction over a million unsolved mysteries. Querulous curiosity creates an existential despair, which intensifies an ongoing dissatisfaction with the petty successes of his pointless life. Not every person can hope to win at the Olympics, charm millions on the screen, or set the fiscal policies of a nation. Both in ordinary life and at the cosmic level, dissatisfaction pursues the skeptic.

In The Conquest of Happiness, Bertrand Russell suggested that happiness may be hard to find in the face of overwhelming calamity. But, that is not quite true. There are many stories of people who have cheerfully marched through the most disastrous situations. Your happiness really does not depend on your circumstances. You have control over it. Whatever is the final story of your life, your epitaph can still be "I did my best and lived a happy life." Happy survival in a harsh environment is a worthy goal. The Intuition Way is a groundbreaking work that challenges our traditional understanding of the meaning of our lives. The Intuition Way offers you new insights from the world of philosophy.

The famed psychiatrist, Frankl, suggested that, even when the world appeared abysmally evil, a purpose was absolutely needed for survival. Having encountered the horrors of the Nazi concentration camps, he lived to narrate the dreaded moment, when a fellow prisoner ceased to struggle for life. Usually, the prisoner refused to go out on to the parade grounds. "He just lay there, hardly moving. No entreaties, no blows, no threats had any effect. He simply gave up. There he remained, lying in his own excreta, and nothing bothered him any more." His system had stopped being driven by a purpose. Such people died soon thereafter. A purpose is needed by the system for survival itself. A purpose enabled survival. Frankl submitted that, despite the capricious torture and beatings, thousands of inmates still did struggle against all odds to eke out a life. They had a purpose in life, whatever it was, which helped them to survive. The machine needs a purpose. But, these need not be large purposes - like having a notable impact on the cosmos. A hope of meeting a son after the war was a purpose. Even a decision to harden oneself against suffering was a sufficient purpose. After the war, Frankl established a major field in psychiatry, assisting thousands of suicidal patients around the world to recover by discovering an acceptable purpose in life.

The Intuition Way is a transformative work that has the potential to change the way you view your life. The 5 steps to freedom still your negative emotions, and the wisdom in the Intuition Way makes you realize that you have to accept life as it comes. You have to discover a purpose and find rewards in your work. If misfortune surrounds you and life appears meaningless, negative emotions can dominate you. Peace of mind and joy in your work are not available off the shelf.

In a world where different political parties suggest different dreams for the world, it can be difficult to know what to aim for. Different political parties often have conflicting visions for the future, which can create conflict and division. This can lead to people feeling hopeless and lost. The ideal answer is for each person to follow his/her own dream. Dreams are important for several reasons. First, they give people hope. When people are feeling hopeless, they are more likely to give up on their goals. Dreams give people something to strive for, even when things are tough. Second, dreams give people a sense of purpose. When people have a dream, they feel like they are part of something bigger than themselves.

They feel like they are making a difference in the world. Third, dreams can help people achieve their goals. When people are focused on their dreams, they are more likely to put in the hard work and dedication necessary to achieve them. We need to create a culture that values dreams and encourages people to pursue them. We need to teach children the importance of dreaming and help them develop their own dreams. We need to eliminate the barriers that prevent people from pursuing their dreams, such as poverty, discrimination, and lack of opportunity. Society needs to encourage people to dream and create a world where people feel safe to pursue their dreams.

Each individual has a special ability. Find the things that you can do effortlessly, which others find difficult. That will be your area of excellence. You also have the capacity to improve any job that you are currently engaged in. When this becomes your focus, any improvement in your performance will become rewarding, filling you with vitality. You will find that even if your life has no meaning, and misfortune surrounds you, focusing on such things will bring you happiness. By following the 5 steps and the practical wisdom in this chapter, the intuition of your prefrontal cortex reveals the truth.

*The Intuition Way is the first book in the world to provide the insightful 20 millisecond intuition/pattern recognition link between events, emotions and motor responses.*

CHAPTER 9

# SOCIAL COMPARISON

*"Comparison is the thief of joy."*
Theodore Roosevelt

Social comparison is a relentless and often troubling drive within you. The Intuition Guide is a must-read for anyone who wants to understand and develop their intuition. It explains subconscious processes that seriously manipulate people without their knowledge. For example, the social comparison drive compares the individual with others and if he is found wanting, triggers pain and makes the individual lash out against another. He does not know why he is behaving badly. The knowledge of this hidden process can liberate the individual and make him free of envy. Self awareness can help you to still the emotional turmoil set off by this incessant subconscious process. Social comparison works both ways. It enables you to fit into the social hierarchy of your community. It enables you to improve your performance through subconscious imitation of the people you admire. Nature even limits the hidden process to a comparison among your equals, creating a realistic potential for improvement.

On the other hand, social comparison triggers a feeling of helplessness and despair about your failure to achieve comparable levels. It generates anger towards your superiors. When you compare yourself with lower levels of society, it initiates the emotions of gratitude and guilt. An acceptance that you are unique, that the wealth, talents and skills of people will always vary can help to still negative feelings related to social comparison. While the subconscious process will work to improve yourself, an awareness of its manipulative workings can help to still your emotional turmoil.

The Social Comparison Theory was initially proposed by social psychologist Leon Festinger in 1954. The theory proposes that individuals have an internal drive to evaluate their own opinions and desires by comparing themselves to others. People look at outside images to evaluate their own views and abilities. These images are sought to be realistic and achievable. The drive to compare reduces as the comparison image diverges from their images of their own views and abilities. People tend to move into groups of similar opinions and abilities, and they move out of groups that fail to satisfy their comparison drive. The theory suggests that while people do improve their abilities through comparison, they do not change their views significantly through the same process.

The social comparison drive became a survival need, when

grazing animals grouped together to protect themselves. The groups moved and acted together, without any overall plan. Unlike an army detachment, which follows an overall plan, individual emotional controls achieve cooperative behavior in herds. Social comparison helped herds to imitate the behavior of equals to choose cooperative patterns of behavior. These tendencies create a status structure of higher and lower groups. A dominance hierarchy is established, with leaders and followers. Each group compare themselves within their own group. At the watering hole, the leader drinks first. Others instinctively follow. Social comparison enabled individual assessments of supportive group behavior.

Without our awareness, our nervous system monitors the behavior of people all around us. If we step into an elevator, our muscles stiffen so as to avoid encroaching into the private territories of others. The formal atmosphere of a museum quiets our conversation. If someone stops in the middle of the street to look up, others will also look up. If someone you respect bows to authority, you are more likely to follow suit. We tend to compare and imitate. We sense their tension and imitate their focus of attention. All this is done without much conscious awareness. Social comparison is a ceaseless part of our subconscious mental processes.

Social comparison is a pattern recognition process, which compares the behavior and achievements of others to assess one's own position in the social group. A person understands his rank in the hierarchy, measured in terms of wealth, official status, or physical prowess. When people are generally comparable, such as in a school yard, behavior patterns decide the hierarchy. Leaders tend to be aggressive, to push back if pressed and to intrude into other's spaces. Anger establishes dominance. Fear subdues the follower. Shame and guilt prevent actions, which are injurious to the herd. The generated emotions continually decide the social structure.

Pattern recognition of comparative behavior triggers emotional control signals, which modify behavior within milliseconds. Within the blink of an eye, your body prepares for an infinite range of variations of the fight, or flight response. Fear, or anger triggers immediate responses. Adrenalin increases. Heart beats increase to improve blood supply. Blood pressure rises and breathing changes. Acidity increases in the stomach. The excretory system prepares to clear toxin. Without your conscious awareness, the comparison process makes you feel fear, guilt, shame, or despair about your comparative stance. These are subtle bodily responses, which manipulate your behavior and disturb your peace of mind.

Hidden social comparison triggers emotional responses. Your conscious awareness of the generated ill feelings follows the process. The experiments of Benjamin Libet uncovered your helpless role in this powerful pattern recognition routine. He. discovered that your motor systems act before you are consciously aware of you choice of action. Your mind processes knowledge faster than your conscious thoughts. Subconscious social comparison may trigger negative emotions like anger, fear, shame, or guilt, or despair. When you feed realistic data to the system you can prevent such emotions from being triggered. Even if bad feelings are triggered, you can quiet them by paying conscious attention to them.

Fortunately, both these actions are within your conscious control. In its intuitive wisdom, a focus of attention on reasonable data will cause your mind to absorb it and to respond reasonably. It will also subdue negative emotions, if you consciously observe them from a distance. You can prevent the emotion from being triggered by changing your attitudes through new knowledge. You can still those emotions by becoming conscious of them when they are triggered.

The social comparison drive evaluates comparisons with perceived equals on the emotional values of material possessions and social relationships. The high appeal of a neighbor's gleaming new car enhances the pain of a missed loan installment on one's own battered jalopy. One's inability to match the achievements of others switches to anger over the unfairness of it all. Anger redirects to the nearest victim. Subconscious social comparison triggers destructive envy, which harms people and makes them wish ill upon their neighbors.

Envy is founded on a wrong view of fairness. A natural sense of fairness makes parents treat their children equally. Our political systems stand for equality. But, life is neither ideal, nor fair. There will always be other people with more talents, more wealth, or more health. Neither is fairness a workable social concept. The brilliant insights of a few stand behind great achievements of man. The inventor of the wheel alone contributed lifetimes of effort to all of humanity. History shows that depriving talented people in the name of fairness leads only to the proven poverty of the socialist systems. Even if it is not fair, society can thrive only if it rewards those who contribute more. Once this reality of the world around us seeps in, envy has no place.

The social comparison drive reduces conflicts in groups. A person, who feels no guilt is likely to harm others and to harm the fabric of society. The so called mirror neuron network enables us to sense the emotional responses of others concerning our errors and omissions. We tend to feel the weight of their contempt or scorn as painful emotions. Eisenberger's research at UCLA confirms activity in the neural pain circuits, when a person suffers social rejection. The system triggered the pain of guilt and shame by comparing selfish behavior with the moral code of the group. Guilt causes a person to express regret and so, he is likely to be forgiven. This reduces the chances of retaliation and consequent conflict. The social comparison drive discourages unsocial actions and compels members to act for group benefit.

The hidden process of social comparison triggers the painful processes of envy. When the achievements of others cause you discomfort, become aware of the negative emotion. Should you suffer the emotions of an animal past? Is the pain of envy justified? Do you not have advantages, which the other lacks? If you fail in one area, can you not discover equally satisfying, but achievable goals elsewhere? Can you not cherish the many advantages that you have in life? Accepting the reality of your own failures will still envy and make you feel a better person. The success of your neighbor will then only inspire you to do better in your own life.

Millions of buying decisions in the market place are triggered through the social comparison process. Fashions change, when role models decide to wear their skirts long, or short. Word of mouth advertising is an acceptance of advantages of a product, as perceived by a friend or neighbor. The gestures of film stars are copied by millions of fans. The mirror neuron network may have roles to play in this process, where motor regions imitate the responses of goal directed actions of another person. Evidently, we will imitate the actions of someone we admire, because our neural network subconsciously decides that an improvement in performance is desirable! We can leave it to nature to subconsciously improve our performance through social comparison!

*The Intuition Way is the first book in the world to provide a comprehensive overview of the 20 millisecond intuition/pattern recognition link between events, emotions, and motor responses.*

# THE CRISIS OF ENVY AND JEALOUSY

*"Envy is the ulcer of the soul." -*
*William Shakespeare*

### *How To Let Go Of Envy And Jealousy*

Overcoming envy and jealousy is a crying need for good natured people, because they feel ashamed of those emotions. Jealousy clearly differs from envy. Jealousy originates from fear or anger over the prospect of failure in achieving a desired goal. Career growth, a partner's love, or a mother's undivided attention are usually the threatened goals. Envy originates from regret, leading to anger, over one's powerlessness to get an alluring asset owned by a perceived equal.

A neighbor's brand new car triggers envy. Jealousy originates from the prospect of failure and envy from actual failure. These distressing human emotions are sad left overs from an animal past. The Intuition Way is a pioneering work that offers a new and real understanding of emotions. When you have such feelings, you can overcome envy and jealousy following the 5 steps in this book and the advice in this chapter. But, if you are a victim of jealousy or envy, your options to escape their ill effects are limited.

Nerve signals trigger a pang of jealousy in Joe, when the boss praises his colleague's report. Those signals originate from neural systems with millions of years of evolutionary history. Those systems , enabled animals to survive in a hostile world. They respond within milliseconds of sensing danger. Within the blink of an eye, the animal's body prepares for fight, or flight. Fear, or anger triggers immediate responses. How can a few words from the boss, or a glimpse of expensive jewelry trigger painful emotions? Nature stores knowledge on an unimaginable scale within your body. Joe's brain stores memories of evolutionary experiences from millions of years.

It remembers his poor marks in school twenty years ago, or the data he overlooked in his report. A word of praise from Joe's boss to his colleague can bring, within milliseconds, images of his weak report and its imagined, or real career consequences. Within that time span his body begins to respond. Joe has no conscious control over the responses of his body. Conscious awareness comes after his mind processes data.

The brilliant experiments of Benjamin Libet uncovered the gulf between motor activity and awareness. He studied subjects who voluntarily pressed a button, while noting the position of a dot on a computer screen, which shifted its position every 43 milliseconds. The noted moment of depressing the button was the moment of conscious awareness; the exact instant the subject thought the button was pressed. Each time, Libet had also timed the beginning of motor neuron activity in the brains of his subjects. He discovered that awareness occurred 350 milliseconds AFTER the beginning of motor activity. Overcoming envy, or jealousy is Joe's task after those emotions have already taken control of his mind.

Jealousy can be both good and bad. Thomas Jefferson believed that it was jealousy, which protected a truly free government and enabled it to prosper. Jealousy is a primary and evolutionary pattern recognition response. Everybody experiences it because of imagined, or real fears. The perennial fear of failure triggers jealousy against perceived rivals in a competitive world. In public life, jealousy increases public vigilance. Romantic jealousy fears abandonment, loss of love, or of being dishonored in a relationship. For valued friendships, jealousy is triggered by the possibility of losing influence or times spent together. Competitive jealousy among siblings constantly causes friction in families. At abnormal levels, extreme insecurity, immaturity, or the tendency to be a "control freak" can trigger morbid, psychotic, pathological, or delusional jealousy.

Jealousy increases awareness and reduces judgment. There is greater awareness of the competitor's actions. Often innocent actions are assumed to contain ulterior motives. A fair judgment of the competitor becomes difficult. A jealous person takes precautionary measures. Fear of a repetition of previous experiences of failure trigger angry and vindictive attacks. Jealousy increases one's sense of insecurity and reduces feelings of self worth, leading to dejection and depression. Sibling jealousy leads to constant fights in families.

Marital jealousy leads to repetitive cycles of violence. A man beats up his wife in a jealous rage. Her pain makes him sorry and he asks for forgiveness. She forgives him and hopes that the gentler phase of their relationship will persist. But, later jealousy attacks again and the cycles of violence continue. Normal sibling rivalry in larger families cause constant bickering between children and strain their weary parents. Jealousy is triggered when the fight for a window seat, or when the choice of a place to eat is lost. While parents can try to be fair, one person has to lose in any choice. The more emotional children are likely to respond with anger, or dejection. Parents should spend one on one time with each child. Consider each incident as an opportunity to make the child learn the concept that life is not fair. It always hands out uneven shares of problems and opportunities. Each child also has her own unique talents and weaknesses.

Unreasonable anger, or self pity will only weaken them in a competitive world. Childhood experiences should lead to maturity, where they learn to cope with their difficulties, while calmly accepting inequality and occasional failures. Problems of marital jealousy are common in the early phases of most marriages. Men who have such problems begin with a low sense of self esteem. Locker room stories of infidelity add to their insecurity. Youthful imagination makes them intensely aware of signals of real or imagined infidelity.

Uncommon jealousy may cause them to call to "check in," or to monitor telephone and address books. After usually groundless probes, men feel ashamed of their behavior and become even more insecure. Such confrontations can lead to increasing cycles of disharmony. A loving partner can assure the man of his innate worth and help him to accept himself as he is. If the man has a degree of self awareness, he can also get over the problem himself. Unfortunately, since self awareness is possible for only for a small group of sensitive people, violently jealous husbands remain an unsolved problem for society.

Some women have the strength of will to respond with self assurance to violence. They can avoid further violence by firmly warning their partner at the outset that violence will immediately end their marriage, or be reported to the police. At the same time, the woman should be vigilant in keeping and maintaining trust and avoid behaviors, which can sow the seeds of suspicion. But, in the vast majority of cases, the victim will be too frightened to take such action. Wherever possible, the victim should speedily seek the assistance of friends, or family to escape from such situations. Sensitive people feel ashamed of feeling jealous, when the boss speaks kindly to a colleague, or when their partner speaks to a friend. An awareness of that discomfort can help you to change your life! The Intuition Way is a must-read for anyone who wants to understand and develop their intuition. Never underestimate the power of these intuition signals. With its vast wisdom, your mind has identified danger to one of your cherished goals. Your discomfort comes, because your mind has already discovered a subconscious weakness. You don't consciously know what it is. Search your mind for the reasons.

Remember that hostility towards a perceived competitor underlies your own fear that you may not achieve your goal. It is not the competitor's faults, but your own weaknesses, which trigger fears and discomfort within you. Search your mind. One of the seemingly innocuous things you recall could be the pivotal underlying problem behind your discomfort. Think about what action you can take. If this new possibility threatens your cherished goal, think whether you can change your goal, or accept the consequences of failure. When you have a plan to deal with the problem, or have accepted the possibility of failure, you will not be troubled by jealousy.

Envy is founded on the wrong premises. Human beings have a sense of fairness. Parents try to treat their children equally and our political systems emphasizes the equality of all people. This sense that we deserve a fair share of things is at the root of envy. Unfortunately, life is not fair. While everybody would like to have equal opportunities and talents, the distribution of benefits is widely distorted. There will always be others with more talents, wealth, or health. Nor is fairness a workable social concept. Human achievements were made possible by the brilliant ideas of a few.

The person, who invented the wheel alone contributed lifetimes of effort to all of humanity. Society needs to reward those who contribute ideas and management skills. History shows that depriving them leads but to the poverty of the socialist systems. Our own prosperity depends on the recognition and reward of talents and responsibilities. Even if it conflicts with our sense of fairness, we need to reconcile ourselves to the idea that a society can thrive only if it rewards those who contribute more. Once this reality of the world around us seeps in, overcoming envy is easier. Envy is an emotion which refuses to accept failure. It makes you feel pain, so that you will do something about it. Triggered by social comparison, the envy drive follows several paths, each path adding to your pain. Envy focuses on your neighbor, triggering sequential visions of her many successes. Each vision will be compared with your failures, intensifying your torment. Envy then adds the pain of guilt, since it is shameful to feel envy. When you remember that her successes are accompanied by problems, envy says "Aw, just sour grapes!" You feel guilty about the need to find "excuses" for your failures. Envy then adds more pain by reminding you that the feeling itself is a sign of failure.

"You are feeling bad, because you failed!" Envy strikes without your conscious awareness. When you feel it, it is already too late! Your mind has begun comparing and the process immediately highlights your failures. Only self awareness can stop these escalating drives. Identifying the emotion as it is triggered can stop the drive in its tracks. Become aware of your habitual patterns of comparison. Recognize the onset of the "Not fair!" feeling. Most people justify their ill will as a fairness issue. The sense of failure triggers anger, which is redirected as anger towards a cruel fate, or an innocent victim. Looking from the outside on those feelings will help to still the emotion. After all, so far, your best efforts have still led to failure. Such failure has to be acknowledged. Such acceptance can help you to still envy. Self awareness will put your prefrontal cortex in charge. Calmly accepting failure, it will make plans for the future. Overcoming envy is a matter of improved self awareness through constant practice! The Intuition Way is a groundbreaking work that will change the way we think about our troubling emotions. The five steps to freedom still the pain of the attacks of envy and jealousy.

The wisdom and scientific evidence in this chapter will convince you that the pain comes from your own perceived failings. You need to come to terms with your pain. The reasons for the pain will not disappear, but accepting the reality of your own failures will still envy and make you feel like a better person. Focus on the positives and the actions you can take. Do you not have advantages that the other person lacks? Can you not do something to win next time? Can you not discover equally satisfying, but achievable goals elsewhere? Can you not cherish the many advantages that you have in life? The success of your neighbor will then only inspire you to do better in your own life. Carry on your life by doing your best, without comparing yourself to others. By following the five steps and absorbing the practical wisdom in this chapter, the intuition of your prefrontal cortex will reveal to you the truth for you to create a bright future.

# THE CRISIS OF BOREDOM

*"There are no uninteresting things,
only uninterested people."*
G.K. Chesterton

### Learn To Be Permanently Rid Of Boredom

The Intuition Way is a transformative work that has the potential to change the way we live our lives. We can eliminate the negatives from our lives! Life should never be boring! There is a lasting cure for boredom, which is, after all, an awful state of mind. You suddenly lack interest in your surroundings and find it difficult to concentrate on anything. Boredom usually happens in three typical situations. You are prevented from doing something you want to do. You are compelled to do a particular job. You simply cannot find anything interesting to do. Your mind recognizes the situation and triggers the boredom emotion. Emotions program your behavior. In the primeval world, emotion signals mechanically modified the behavior of animals to enable their survival.

Anger made an animal fight, fear caused it to flee, and boredom made it abandon unprofitable efforts and search for more urgent survival tasks. Emotions generated programmed responses for a primitive world. But now, events move at a slower pace. The immediate demands of life are not so compellingly urgent. Today, being calm and composed is useful, and patience is a necessary virtue. But sadly, primitive animal emotions still work their ancient logic. They impose harmful behavioral patterns. Boredom dumps you into an awful level of consciousness. It creates anxiety about not doing anything. Boredom poses greater risks of developing depression and drug or alcohol addiction. Bored people display anger, aggressive behavior, and exhibit weak interpersonal skills. They do poorly at work and at school. The permanent cure for boredom begins with the awareness that you can be comfortable with longer periods of stillness. Know that boredom is a manipulative action by the primitive part of your mind, and self-awareness can be used to switch it off.

You have joined one of those long, tiresome queues. Usually, people bring along something to read, play Nintendo, or watch others to avoid boredom. But you don't need such crutches. It is possible to avoid feeling bored altogether. Imagine Buddhist monks, who sit quietly for hours while they meditate. They have found a cure for boredom. In the stillness of the prefrontal cortex, your rational brain, there is actually no space for boredom!

Mental fatigue can be caused by repetitive tasks. Boredom in such a situation is understandable. But feeling that a task is too hard or too easy is only an excuse. In the real world, there is no task that is not substantially repetitive and tiresome. An accountant for a multinational corporation repeats many procedures over the years. A software architect pores over an infinity of details. Even the President of a country sits for hours listening to monotonous speeches and reports. In every field, there are people who cope successfully with such situations. If you feel weary about such situations, remember, there is a cure for boredom. There are times, when a news item, or a movie scene grabs your attention and keeps you absorbed. But, have you not kept switching channels on TV, to find nothing interesting? Even the replay of a favorite movie feels boring and uninteresting. It is important to realize that you are being manipulated by your nervous system. The restlessness and lack of interest are the effects of programmed emotional signals. Once you have learned the simple cure for boredom, your mind will find so many interesting things to attend to.

There are people who enjoy even the most repetitive assembly line work, and others who maintain a steadily depressed attitude to life and complain bitterly of monotony even on the most varied work. It is the attitude, and not the work, that makes the difference. The first cure for boredom is the realization that it is not the situation, but an emotion, which is acting up within you. An emotion envelops you in its level of consciousness. Your nervous system has succeeded over millions of years by routinely focusing all available resources on a single objective. Fear compels you to escape, without being tempted to stay back and fight. So, also, when you are bored, the system inhibits pleasant memories and colors the situation bleak. The system is manipulating you.

Your mind contains a prefrontal cortex, a rational part of your brain that views any situation with equanimity. It evaluates the world without emotions. Imagine a computer printout of your boring situation. You are waiting in line, doing a repetitive task, or trying to find something to do. It is just another thing you do in life. It can be viewed as a situation in life, not a tiresome situation. A neutral view is the view of the prefrontal cortex. The 5 steps to freedom in this book can activate the prefrontal cortex and your viewpoint will instantly change. You will immediately feel that it is perfectly okay to be doing nothing. Boredom takes control within a few milliseconds. You are in a darkened lecture hall. Before you know it, time seems to hang heavily. You cannot focus on the slides and the drone of voices. You become bored, impatient, and restless. Such emotions take control because you are merely a troubled spectator, watching the habitual thought patterns of your emotional brain. One of the 5 steps, self-awareness, activates the prefrontal cortex, which can instantly quell boredom. When the prefrontal cortex becomes aware of the physical symptoms of engulfing boredom, the emotion itself will become disconnected and vanish. When equilibrium is reached, the prefrontal cortex, your common sense, will take control. You will reach a stage where a quiet peace surrounds you. Then you can focus on anything of interest. At a lecture, focus on constructively criticizing the speaker.

Controlling the focus of your mind provides a lasting cure for boredom. Mindfulness courses have improved the performance of novice meditators on tasks of sustained attention and working memory. They were also less depressed than those who did not receive such training. The pattern-sensing logic of the mind works to quell boredom and change attitudes. It does take a little practice to become so self-aware. But imagine the benefits of being free of boredom for the rest of your life!

Philosophers have written that the experience of boredom is an indication that nature has not served its purpose of making life worth living. But, they did not realize that boredom is an emotion evolved to keep animals focused on profitable efforts. But, with your prefrontal cortex level of consciousness, you have no need to be so manipulated by your nervous system. The Intuition Way is a must-read for anyone who wants to understand the power of intuition and how to use it to their advantage. When boredom has been overcome, prefrontal cortex will also find many ways to keep your mind occupied. Reduced reported levels of boredom were considered reliable indicators of whether treated drug addicts would stay clean. Long distance drivers, who reported little boredom, played mental games, such as counting of passing objects. They were also safer drivers. Just self awareness can set you free. A freed prefrontal cortex can develop new skills and hobbies. Freed from boredom, your own patterns sensing mechanisms will find joy in the beauty of the world around you.

The Intuition Way provides a fresh and insightful look at how your mind works. The 5 steps to freedom still your negative emotions, and the restlessness and discomfort disappear. The wisdom in the book makes you realize that boredom is merely an emotion. When emotions are stilled, the background chatter vanishes. By stilling our emotions, we free ourselves. We are freed from the prejudices of our social group, the painful startle responses, the needless guilt, the glancing over our shoulder for competitors, the limitations in our life, the put downs and insults, the greed, the dissatisfaction, and the disappointments. As the primitive attacks of fear, resentment, and anger reduce, and boredom disappears, our intuition will trigger joy, wonder, and gratitude. We will be able to see the world from a clear and objective mind, and we will be able to enjoy the sunset because we are not bored.

*The Intuition Way is the first book in the world to provide the insightful 20 millisecond intuition/pattern recognition link between events, emotions and motor responses.*

# CHAPTER 12

## THE. CRISIS OF SADNESS

*"Sadness is like a cloud. It won't last forever."*
Paulo Coelho

### Learn To Accept The Loss

The Intuition Way is a groundbreaking work that will change the way we think about emotions. Emotions rule your lower level instinctual intelligences, which propose survival strategies for your life. The 5 steps given in the book and an understanding of the logic of the evolutionary triggers of emotions can help you deal with troubling issues. I am so sad - those words cry out for help. The feelings they express do not refer to a mild, momentary unhappiness, but more to the intense grief, caused by a loss, or a disappointment. The feeling does not come just from frustration, which can make you feel persistently gloomy, or dejected. Nor does it come from a sense of futility, which can trigger a mood of brooding despondency or depression. Sadness essentially deals with a sense of irreparable loss over "what might have been."

The loss casts a pall over every vista. Like the pain of loss of a limb, the feeling irretrievably touches primary aspects of your life. Those words also express a cry for help. The sad person suffers. You feel empty or numb. You may cry a lot. It may affect your sleep. You may eat too little, or too much. The sadness takes away your energy and makes you feel more tired. Some people even get stomach aches and headaches. The emotion makes it difficult for you to focus on your work. So, your output suffers. You may spend less time with friends and even find it difficult to concentrate on reading, or on watching TV. Sadness affects your work, your health and even prevents you from enjoying even the smallest pleasures in life.

The emotion can be triggered for any number of reasons. It could be the loss of a loved one, or a divorce. A disappointment, which changes your expectations from life can be the cause. You may have regrets about things you did, or did not do. You may have moved away from a town, away from friends and relatives, who gave you comfort. Needless tensions created by family or teenagers could cause you to painfully miss a happier life.

Pain or suffering for a loved one could cause the sadness. In every case, the recalled images of "what life might have been" cause distress. It is quite normal for you to feel intense grief over a loss, or disappointment. But time is a great healer. However deep your grief, the sorrow will reduce over a period of days, or months. This is a normal neural event. It is a part of the design of nature. Nerve impulses tend to fade over time. The emotional signals, which caused you distress will fade over time, unless your own thoughts prevent the healing process. Normally, a wound also heals gradually. But, if you keep irritating it, it will remain raw and painful. Repeated living over your pain and loss will intensify the neural patterns. New "speed dial circuits" will be created within the nervous system, which continue to trigger the same level of distress. The pain will refuse to go away.

One day, you must move on. Sadness heals. It is an emotion, which helps you to deal with sudden loss. Crying softens painful memories. Reliving the experiences help you to adjust to a new painful reality. Upto a point. If the sadness persists and causes you continuing distress, you must act to deal with it. You have to become convinced that it is time to leave the painful past behind and bring back your peace of mind. After all, it affects your work and your health. It prevents you from getting on with the rest of your life. The 5 steps in the book will only succeed if you are convinced that they are necessary. Are you prepared to move on? There are avenues of thought, which reinforce the pain pathways. A loss implies an irreversible change in your life. Instead of moving on with your life, you keep thinking about what might have been. The recall of a beloved image, which is no more possible will create fresh pain.

Guilt also plays a part. A sense of loyalty towards the absent relationship could keep you from thinking of a happy life alone. Your mind will shut away such thoughts with a sense of guilt. Guilt is the second emotion, which will reopen the wound. Out of the same sense of loyalty you may feel that sadness is justified and keep dwelling within the emotion. Reliving the past and feeling guilty about moving on will both keep the pain both fresh and raw. Your common sense is a rigorously independent intelligence within your nervous system. Within your triune brain, it is a powerful prefrontal network, which can be induced to take charge of your thought processes. Anger causes an animal to attack. Fear causes it to run away. And sadness causes it to withdraw from activity and adjust to loss. Emotions are triggered by neural signals in the limbic system. But, those signals can go haywire. While emotions serve a purpose, erratic speed dial circuits can cause particular emotions to unreasonably dominate your behavior. Fear, anger, or sadness can overwhelm you. If these circuits have not attained abnormal dominance (requiring medical treatment), the attention of your common sense can still the troubling emotions initiated by them.

Your common sense can act only if your mind is not dominated by your emotions. In the first place, you need to deal with your sense of guilt. Guilt plays an important role in group behavior, preventing you from actions, which would trouble your community. Apply your common sense to reduce your pangs of guilt. Self awareness has that effect. Your problem is not "I am sad," but "I am so sad." You are suffering too much. Become aware of your guilt feelings about not dwelling on sad memories, or even on moments of joy after a bereavement.

Pay attention to the physical symptoms of your feelings. Your attention to the physical symptoms will still the pangs of guilt. While sadness is justified, your common sense will know that excessive sadness is not a reasonable emotion. You will know that you must get on with your life. Your common sense will tell you. All you need is self awareness.

You also need to realign your world view. It is but human to have something to look forward to - a happy plan for your life. Sadness intrudes, when that plan has irrevocably changed for the worse. You will not, ever again, share your burdens, your joys and sorrows with your loved one. Or, in a crucial disappointment, your career has changed for the worse. It is a situation, where every context reminds you of your loss. Your subconscious mind will cope with this situation only if you develop a new plan for your life. This is a new stage in your life. Think creatively of how you can make your life meaningful again. The very decision to plan a new beginning will suddenly open your horizons to fresh view points.

Instead of dwelling on the "what might have been" images, which cause you distress, you will open your eyes to the world again. Even as you work on a revised plan for your life, you will constantly encounter the "what might have been" images all around you. They will repeatedly trigger the sadness emotion. Become aware of the physical symptoms of that emotion. It could be a pang in your chest, or a knot in your stomach. It may be a drive, which makes you want to cry. Emotions are neural signals, with distinct symptoms. They will lose their power to dominate you, when you pay attention to the symptoms. Your common sense will realize that your feelings are not overpowering world views, but simple physical symptoms. Over a period of time, the emotion will have been stilled.

When people experience sadness over long periods, their facial muscles slowly adjust to meet the dominant emotion. People will say "There is a sadness in her eyes." Your facial expressions can induce emotions. Try this experiment. Glare at this page and say "Stop it!" You will notice that your voice takes on a sharper tone. Great actors feel the emotion of a hero by copying facial expressions. Become aware of your facial expressions. Practice a more cheerful expression. While it may feel stupid at the beginning, your facial muscles will adjust and you will discover that your mind will also act in context to bring you more cheerful thoughts. Does your sadness persist because of drugs, medication, or alcohol? Is it caused by changes in hormone levels? If there is no clear cause for your sadness, see if sunshine, music, or friends can cheer you up. A good night's rest alone may cheer you up. Ordinary sad patches will clear in a few days. If your sadness persists without a significant cause for more that two weeks, check with your doctor. A deeper and more intense sadness, without a clear cause may be a depression. If it seriously affects your life, seek professional counsel.

CHAPTER 13

# THE CRISIS OF FEAR

*"The only way to defeat fear
is to face it head-on."*
*Eleanor Roosevelt*

### How To Face Your Fears

The Intuition Way is unique in providing a comprehensive overview of the 20-millisecond intuition/pattern recognition link between events, emotions, and motor responses. Recognition of the potential for pain or an unrecognizable event causes fear. The amygdalae, organs in the limbic system, detect such possibilities and send the signals that generate the fear emotion. The anger emotion switches on attitudes and behaviors that support confrontation. Fear, on the other hand, responds to danger by recalling fearful images, preparing the body for flight, and signaling muscles to freeze or flee. These events occur in milliseconds.

Fear acts instantly. It will stiffen your muscles before you can walk to the edge of a precipice. While fear signals act swiftly to avoid danger, they intensify when danger is unavoidable. In such situations, fear signals inhibit conscious thinking and set off subconscious searches for escape routes while preparing the body to freeze, flee, or defend itself. Those subconscious searches flash images of the results of failure. A lack of escape avenues intensifies the fearful emotion. Together, the recalled images, the urges to escape, and the bodily preparations for stress feel unpleasant.

During the early beginnings of life, nature developed the amygdalae as special-purpose organs in the brain to remember and respond to danger signals. They become sensitive to sensory signals that accompany past painful events. Such sensitivity in the amygdalae of animals has been extensively verified. In typical experiments, a rat is exposed to a painful foot shock accompanied by a sound. Later, when the sound alone is heard, the amygdalae will fire fear signals. Such painful experiences were seen to develop "speed dial (LTP) circuits," which later responded instantly to the related sound signal. The organs became oversensitive to such signals. As essential as the vertebrae, these organs were early components of the brains of fish, amphibians, reptiles, birds, and mammals. As the primary defense response mechanism, the amygdalae recognized danger patterns and impelled animals to fight, freeze, or escape.

Fear is expressed at increasing levels as worry, anxiety, dread, terror, and panic. These levels are determined by the imminence of danger. Worry and anxiety are triggered by the anticipation of being harmed in the future. Dread, terror, and panic concern the immediate present. At the highest levels, terror and panic overwhelm people, causing them to make irrational choices. While terror is an apprehension of impending danger, horror is a sickening and painful experience. Horror is the emotion that lays the foundations for the amygdala to sense the background of painful events.

The amygdalae remember the images, sounds, words, and situations that accompanied the horror of injury, ridicule, social rejection, loss of loved ones, or career failure. Subsequently, the detection of any related signals triggers fear, often without the person knowing the cause of her fear. These events occur in less time than the 300 millisecond time span it takes for consciousness to be aware of them. On receiving fear signals from the amygdalae, the hypothalamus acts reflexively to control the reproductive, vegetative, endocrine, hormonal, visceral, and autonomic functions of the body. Breathing, digestion, blood circulation, brain activity, and body fluid flows are instantly affected. The signals from the amygdalae dilate the pupils and increase brain wave frequency. They make hair stand on end. They reduce saliva, drying the mouth. They cause sweating and a decrease in skin resistance. They decrease peripheral blood flow and cause hands to become cold. The signals speed breathing and dilate the bronchial tubes to allow more air to reach the lungs. They tighten stomach muscles, slow digestion, and close down the excretory system. They increase the acids in the stomach, causing diarrhea.

The signals travel to the adrenal gland, which produces cortisol, causing an increase in glucose production to provide additional fuel for the muscles and brain to deal with the potential stress. The signals increase blood pressure, release sugar into the blood, and increase the tendency for blood clotting. The signals increase red blood cells. They tense postural muscles, causing hand and body tremors. They dilate blood vessels in skeletal muscles to allow greater blood flow. They slow the functioning of the immune system. The amygdalae trigger a chain of biological events and engulf the mind in the fear emotion, even before the conscious mind can assess the situation. In the modern world, such persistent fear signals are not set off by real physical danger. They are triggered by an instinctive brain, which tries to overcome social and career issues by foolishly preparing the body to freeze, flee, or defend itself. A persistent lack of escape routes from danger leads to the insistent fear signals of anxiety, which raise heart rate and blood pressure over time. Such conditions are believed to lead to heart palpitations, fatigue, nausea, chest pain, shortness of breath, stomach aches, or headaches. Escalating fear signals trigger panic attacks, which have indications similar to the symptoms of heart attacks. Over the years, anxiety has been linked to health issues including arthritis, migraines, allergies, stomach ulcers, and thyroid disease.

The amygdala triggers fear signals, which drive you to escape from danger. It responds to three types of events. The first inherited set of circuits fires on identifying historically harmful events. The second group of neurons develops LTP circuits, which learn to fire upon identifying events that accompany painful experiences. The last group of circuits triggers fear when the system is unable to identify the impact of an event. Over millions of years, nature has assembled in the amygdala a memory for harmful events. Upon recognizing signals of such events, the amygdala instinctively responds by triggering fear. So, most people have an inherited fear of falling, of being suffocated in enclosed spaces, of drowning in water, and of being attacked by rats, cockroaches, or snakes. Even stage fright and a fear of public speaking originate from an instinctive fear of becoming the focus of predators attention. The fear responses of the amygdala to such events are often accompanied by the startle response.

Over a lifetime, the amygdala builds additional sensitivity to pain experiences. Pain may have been caused by physical injury, painful confrontations, the loss of loved ones, a loss of social status, or social rejection. Mirror neurons also trigger pain within us when we see the painful experiences of others. Whenever such pain has been experienced, the amygdala stores memories of the related sensory signals. The Intuition Way is unique in the world in presenting a comprehensive overview of the 20 millisecond link between events, emotions, and motor responses. Fear can be triggered by the fleeting image of an angry face. People suffer from fears of failing, of being ridiculed, and of the loss of loved ones. If a person suffered trauma when left alone as a child, she may fear loneliness.

The human mind recognizes the impact of an event in less than 300 milliseconds. Fear is triggered by the amygdala, when the system is unable to identify the significance of an event. Without the actual experience of such events, people fear death, nuclear war, terrorism, or even threatened changes in their work environments. When fear envelops you for a reason you are unable to fathom, it is useful to list the issues that bother you. You will find that locating the cause of such fear and facing it will free you from the emotion. Fear begins with the startle response. It is the fastest (20 milliseconds) response of the mind to danger through a direct amygdala fear pathway, as reported by Joseph E. LeDoux. He identified a second route (300 milliseconds) through the reasoning processes of the cortex, which can still lead to a sudden onset of fear. Mere movements, sounds, or images can trigger the fearful startle response. The reflex is present at birth. The Intuition Way is unique in the world in suggesting a sweeping pattern recognition logic for such events.

When a newborn senses the possibility of falling, her back arches and her arms and legs flail out. Doctors test the reflex to be sure of an infant's nervous system by simulating a sense of falling by allowing its head to drop slightly. The startle signals from the amygdala activate the sympathetic system, which heightens emotional arousal. Later, the cortical signals may energize the parasympathetic system, dampening emotional tension. Unthinking fear set off by the startle response may be stilled by the reasoned cortical signals, such as when a coiled snake is identified to be just a garden hose. While physical danger was always present in the primitive world, it is less relevant today. Unfortunately, while justified by a tiger in the vicinity, fear responses are unsuitable and unhealthy for a person facing career problems. The possibility of dismissal from work requires a calm and collected reaction. Fear triggers images of unpaid bills and sets off a tightness in your chest, which serves no useful purpose. If a solution to the problem was available to you, you would immediately know it. Worry and anxiety set off by fear rarely find solutions but affect your health. Except for avoiding sudden physical injury, fear is an irrelevant animal response. The cause of such fear is a primitive neural signal from the amygdala, which can be stilled through the practice of self-awareness.

In the instant in which an animal senses danger, its mind identifies a course of action—possibly to slip under a rock. Fear is a creative process that subconsciously searches your mind for ways to escape pain. Your impulsive decisions, when triggered by fear, may not present you with any conscious awareness of the particular pain that you wish to avoid. Pain is triggered by many social emotions, including sadness, disgust, contempt, embarrassment, guilt, and shame. A fear of being ridiculed can make a person decide not to take part in conversation. Fear of experiencing the fear emotion may make a person avoid challenging assignments.

Fear is triggered within the amygdala because its nerve junctions develop special sensitivity to particular sensory signals. Even faint sounds may trigger unbearable fear reactions for patients suffering from post-traumatic stress syndrome. Richard Huganir discovered that timely manipulation of specific molecules that regulate synaptic plasticity in the amygdalae of animals can remove the fear response. He identified an unusual protein that appeared in the amygdala of animals and had been conditioned to respond to sounds accompanying a foot shock. That molecule, which remained for only a few days, appeared to strengthen the fear circuits in the amygdalae. When the researchers eliminated the protein during this period, the animals permanently lost those fear-induced memories. A combination of behavioral and pharmacological therapies aimed at those molecular targets may one day be used to help patients. Scientists from Zurich also found that the hormone oxytocin, related to stress and sex, also reduced amygdala activity.

Self-awareness can reduce the causes of fear. The intense activity in the amygdalae, which causes the fear experience, can be reduced by the attention center of the brain, the rostral anterior cingulate cortex (rACC). Columbia University researchers observed that when fear stimuli were perceived consciously, rACC acted to dampen amygdala activity. The 5 steps in the Intuition Way can make the global effect of fear visible and reduce its impact. For normal people, conscious awareness and acceptance of the fear experience will still stimulate the amygdala. With the conviction that fearlessness can become an acquired habit, the practice of self-awareness can bring a calm and still mind.

Creative management requires alertness, not fear. Fear tends to paralyze. Every vista appears dangerous and threatening. In any threatening situation, you can only do one of three things. Do something about it, avoid it, or live with it. A quiet evaluation will define your response and quiet the fear. The awareness of danger will still be present. Common sense appears when fear is calmed. It is the ability to take calculated risks that makes a project successful. Emotions can also be harmful. When they are not managed properly, they can lead to irrational decisions and behaviors. However, this does not mean that we should avoid emotions altogether. Instead, we should learn to manage our emotions in a healthy way. The way to do this is to accept our emotions. When we deny our emotions, they only become stronger. However, when we accept our emotions, we can begin to understand them and to manage them in a healthy way. The Intuition Way is the only book in the world to provide you with an in-depth awareness of the neural mechanisms that trigger your emotions.

*The Intuition Way is the first book in the world to provide the insightful 20 millisecond intuition/pattern recognition link between events, emotions and motor responses.*

CHAPTER 14

# THE CRISIS OF REVENGE

*"Forgiveness is the key that unlocks
the door of resentment and sets us free."*
Catherine Pulsifer

### How To Develop The Gift Of Forgiveness

The Intuition Way gives you a thorough rundown of emotional traps and aids in your understanding of the evolutionary causes for their occurrence. Resentment and guilt are stilled by forgiveness, which gives common sense the upper hand. Fair judgment is made possible by forgiving others and letting go of small-minded animosity. The crippling ache of guilt is removed from the psyche by forgiveness toward oneself. Guilt and resentment act like a bird flapping in vain against its cage. The abnormal yells and squeals of the brain's basic regions in response to undesirable circumstances are known as emotions. The act of forgiveness calms those areas. The true act of forgiveness removes resentment, bitterness, and guilt from the subconscious mind. Numerous studies show that people who forgive are happier and healthier than those who hold resentments. When troubling visceral responses, which accompany bitterness, resentment, and guilt, are stilled, calm and compassionate views of the world emerge, enabling wiser decision-making. The positive benefits of forgiveness have been seen to be similar whether they are based on religious or secular counseling.

A Gallup Poll in 1988 found that, while 94% said it was important to forgive, 85% felt they needed outside help to be able to forgive. Communities resent people who lie, steal, cheat, sell out, or betray their own values since they threaten everyone. Guilt is also subconsciously triggered when a person acts against accepted social norms. People fear that if they still feel anger or guilt, they will not act to rectify the wrong. They fear that forgiveness could be seen as weakness. The fear of docile acceptance of evil makes it difficult to forgive. Both forgiving an offense and forgiving oneself for wrongdoing feel instinctively wrong because of a false impression of the psychological process of forgiveness. It is not the submissive acceptance of wrongdoing. It is an internal stilling process, not a condonation of evil. It is about stopping inner accusations and complaints. Stilling mental turmoil creates the ability to look calmly at the offense. Such calming exercises are difficult for ordinary people.

Forgiveness is needed because resentment and guilt are the sterile responses of your mind to harmful events. Such responses are triggered by the most primitive parts of your "triune" brain. Within the brain, three evolutionary intelligences compete for control. At the lowest level, a reptilian brain produces territorial responses like anger or raw fear. At the next level, a mammalian brain controls the system through social emotions like guilt and shame. These are the more primitive responses, which have a hapless way of taking charge of your mind. It is within your power to free your mind by stilling such negative emotions. When the mind becomes still, a highly developed human-level brain in the prefrontal regions switches in to make a rational interpretation of your world. With your primitive responses stilled, your compassionate common sense takes control. Forgiveness is its natural state, when negative emotions are stilled. There are simple routines that can still the mind and create conditions where forgiveness takes charge. Resentment and guilt are triggered by subconscious search drives that seek vengeance or to avoid social disapproval.

Such searches go on while you look at a lunch menu or chat with your friend. But when those inner searches encounter the painful results of failure, visceral reactions hit you. You may not even be aware of the cause of your discomfort. The 5 steps in the book provide exercises for relaxing your body so that negative emotions cannot take hold. These exercises can disperse the adrenal hormone cortisol, which supports the fight or flight response, including an increased heart rate. Self-awareness, which requires practice, can identify the physical symptoms of resentment or guilt, instantly stilling the emotions. That leads to the sudden appearance of a surprisingly calm viewpoint. While the 5 steps in the book present one way of achieving forgiveness, the remainder of this chapter deals with the psychology of forgiveness. First, a person can forgive another for a perceived offense. In this case, forgiveness stops resentment and the vindictive drive to inflict punishment.

As Jean Safer suggests, it is not necessary to feel okay about terrible things. Psychological forgiveness is not a process that halts the operation of normal justice. After discarding vindictive resentment, calm and compassionate steps should be taken to prevent the recurrence of such incidents, even if it requires punishment. Forgiveness is the process of replacing subconscious bitterness and resentment with compassionate common sense. That is not a piece of mental acrobatics, but a process achieved through relaxation and self-awareness.

Second, a person may seek forgiveness for an offense committed against another. Forgiveness is not a process of achieving goodwill from the victim. Neither is it a matter of seeking divine pardon. Forgiveness of offenses without a change in behavior by the offender leads only to destructive relationships. Self-forgiveness is about making the decision to atone for the offense while still feeling a humiliating sense of guilt. It is a common-sense admission of having committed an offense, with a calm determination to change. Stilling self-punishing guilt feelings is the same self-awareness process that enables common sense to take control. A conscious decision to forgive may or may not result in the disappearance of resentment over the commitment of an offense by another. Such a decision may be more effective if one feels it to be an act of virtue. The satisfaction of virtue may cause the mind to avoid reliving the issue with resentment. This virtuous satisfaction may increase if the offender persists with the offense. In such cases, virtue becomes a failing.

A virtuous approach may cause subconscious anger to pile up and explode into view against an innocent victim. By permitting someone to persistently break the bounds of courtesy, the virtuous person is also damaging society. The offender will harm others too. It is equally the duty of the virtuous person to prevent or avoid becoming a victim of future offenses. This may be impossible in many cases, particularly when the offenders are in positions of power. The satisfaction of being virtuous or a conscious resignation to the situation will both be equally effective in such situations. Christianity believes that a key divine quality is forgiveness. Such forgiveness requires the believer to forgive his brother. Protestant denominations suggest that divine forgiveness requires a sincere expression of repentance. Even a gift at the altar should be offered only after forgiving others. Acts of penance mediated by the church can also bring divine forgiveness for the Catholic Church. The grant of such divine forgiveness is formally expressed through ritual acts by the church.

In Judaism, a person cannot obtain divine forgiveness for wrongs they have done to others. It is the responsibility of the wrongdoer to recognize their wrongdoing and to seek forgiveness from those who have been harmed. A person can only obtain divine forgiveness for acts against God. Just prior to Yom Kippur, Jews will ask forgiveness of those they have wronged.

On the day itself, they fast and pray for divine forgiveness. For Islam, divinity is the source of all forgiveness. One must ask for divine forgiveness through repentance. In the case of human forgiveness, it is important to both forgive and to be forgiven. In Buddhism, forgiveness is seen as a practice to prevent harmful emotions from creating havoc with one's sense of well-being. Since feelings of hatred and ill-will leave a lasting effect on the mind, forgiveness encourages the cultivation of wholesome emotions. They consider the offender to be the most unfortunate of all and require compassion.

Everett L. Worthington recommends decisional and emotional forgiveness. A decision not to seek revenge or avoid the person reduces the stress. But the objective should be to replace resentment, bitterness, hostility, hatred, anger, and fear with love, compassion, sympathy, and empathy. This prevents subconscious obsessions about the wrong done to you. This can lead to anxiety, depression, and even hives. Worthington has devised a 5-step program called REACH to achieve emotional forgiveness. First, recall the hurt objectively, without blame or self-victimization. Then, empathize by trying to imagine the viewpoint of the person who wronged you. After that, altruism involves experiencing the feeling of being forgiven by someone else. This is followed by a commitment to forgiveness and holding on to forgiveness. The self-awareness suggested on this website enables the prefrontal regions to look calmly at the hurt. Empathy is the process of experiencing the emotions of the offender.

This process may not have a calming effect. Rather than empathy, a common-sense view of the twisted logic of the offender can enable the acceptance of reality - the world as it really is, with all its sores and warts. Self-awareness enables this. The experience of being forgiven by another is a valuable reinforcement of forgiveness. Constant self-awareness and the ability to identify the emotion at its inception are requirements to prevent a recurrence of resentment and guilt.

*The Intuition Way is the first book in the world to provide the insightful 20 millisecond intuition/pattern recognition link between events, emotions and motor responses.*

CHAPTER 15

# THE CRISIS OF INGRATITUDE

*"When you are grateful, fear disappears
and abundance appears."*
Anthony Robbins

### Enjoy The Gift Of Gratitude

Science accepts the unique power of gratitude for good. A sense of gratitude to the Creator is central to Western religion. Those who feel more grateful for the benefits they experience clearly enjoy a better quality of life. But is a sense of gratitude for life justified? With starving children, painful diseases, famines, and earthquakes, how can anyone feel thankful for being thrust into this unforgiving world? For many pessimists, gratitude is a mystifying concept. Even if they are individually and uniquely blessed, can the misery of legions of unfortunates be ignored? For those despairing skeptics, gratitude for life sounds absurd. But those unhappy few are mistaken. They don't need to struggle to feel grateful for life. They will naturally feel grateful and enjoy the celebrated feeling of abundance when they abandon a few misconceptions. It is true that it is hard to break out of old and negative ways of thinking, but it can be done. An escape from despair begins with an insight into why gratitude is reasonable. Then they need to work on losing their feelings of despair. Freed from emotional turmoil, mindfulness living will reveal the wonder of life, despite all its misery. Then the reason for gratitude will become obvious, and its power will change their lives.

Gratitude is essentially an emotion that improves people's behavior. Cynics allege that gratitude changes behavior in expectation of future favors. That is not true. The prospect of future benefits triggers only fearful flattery. Gratefulness is not crafty and does not fawn. Gratitude is a positive emotion filled with goodwill. It acknowledges receiving something valuable, which a person cannot justly claim to deserve. If something is expected in return, the recipient only feels indebted, leading to more avoidance of the giver. Gratitude arises when the recipient feels that nothing is expected in return. It motivates the recipient to have positive and helpful feelings towards the giver.

Gratitude evolved as a social instinct. Animals that live together in herds survive better than loners. Evolution developed specific patterns of social rewards and punishments for the survival of herds. At the highest level, the individual is rewarded with maximal respect and admiration for those heroic actions that benefit the whole herd. For individual interactions, there are persistent and strict codes that deliver reciprocal rewards. An action that benefits the recipient but is costly to the performer fills the recipient with goodwill, motivating a strong desire to return the favor. Harmful actions invite retribution, discouraging unsocial behavior. Invariably, there is a time lag between giving and receiving.

The related emotions persist within the neural network for a reasonable period and subside only when favors or punishments of equal value are delivered to the giver. The emotions of gratitude and revenge implemented those social rules, which ultimately resulted in the domination of all life by herds. Emotions are neural processes that control attitudes and behaviors. An emotion can fill you with terror and even freeze your ability to take a single step. Without that emotion in control, walking is deceptively easy. But fear will freeze you into immobility if you suddenly need to step on a plank a hundred feet above the ground. That fear is not your choice.

You may not even be aware that it has taken control. You will only know the reason why you are afraid. Fear can also be induced by electrical excitation of certain parts of the temporal lobe. Negative and positive emotions originate as distinctive patterns of nerve impulses, which also trigger neurochemical events. They have the capacity to micromanage the fluidity of your muscle movements, your thoughts, your facial expressions, and the choice and tone of your words.

When a positive emotion is experienced, the system releases the neuromodulator dopamine. Dopamine provides clarity for immediate objectives and makes a person feel more energetic and elated. A person feels more aware of and interested in the tasks at hand. Gratitude is a positive emotion that grants a person a powerful sense of well-being.

Gratitude flows from a feeling that life is good. Science discovered that, when you experience the emotion, you will have a sense of well-being. Your health will be better, and you will have a more cheerful attitude toward life. People who experience gratitude sleep better and have more positive thoughts. They face problems well and are more in control of their lives. They cope better with transitions in life. Experiencing gratitude is a true indication of coping well with life. Gratitude works positively. In fMRI studies, the ventromedial prefrontal regions are activated for rewards such as food, money, or pleasant music. Tricomi of Caltech tested subjects, selectively rewarding groups for winning simple games. Subjects with high scores felt comparatively wealthy. Feeling that they had received more than their fair share made them feel grateful. Such subjects showed activation of the ventromedial prefrontal regions indicating pleasure, even when another participant with a low score received a reward. Gratitude makes one feel generous towards weaker members of the group. A feeling that one has more than a fair share triggers gratitude, making a person more generous.

A sense of fairness is subjective. Gratitude can be felt in many aspects of life. Gratitude can be felt about the people who surround you, the things you own, your experience of the present moment, the wonder of life, in comparisons with others, and about your relationship to the cosmos. When enjoying identical benefits, people differ in their assessment of the value, cost, and benevolent intentions of the giver. They feel differing levels of gratitude after being helped. Some may only feel dissatisfaction and resentment. The more fortunate ones enjoy the feeling of gratitude more frequently and in more areas. Science has discovered that people who feel gratitude more often are better adjusted and happier. A sense of well-being indicates the true power of gratitude to modify attitudes.

Gratitude cannot be willed into existence. Gratitude for life can only come from a positive existential position. Gratitude ultimately results from an informed assessment by a person's mind that, in spite of myriad problems, its essential wonder makes life worth living. Such an assessment follows an evaluation of the positives and negatives in one's life. Damasio proposed an evaluation of the "somatic markers" (a store of all reward and punishment-associated experiences) for decision-making by the mind.

The Intuition Way offers a unique and innovative perspective on an intuitive decision-making process where the feedback and feed-forward circuits in the limbic system evaluate all decision parameters, including emotions, to instantly deliver a final decision. Intuition is a miracle of nature with many weaknesses. In the end, each individual weighs despair and boredom against wonder and love to measure the quality of his own life. For the despairing, life is a stupid mistake. To the child, it is a world of joy. By stilling negative emotions, a person can tilt the balance and enjoy the power of gratitude. In the judgment of the mind, good feelings have to be stronger than the negative emotions to feel gratitude. No living person is free from problems in life.

A few are troubled by more than their share and a few others burdened by a negative attitude, which casts a fearsome visage on existence itself. At the same time, there are happy and cheerful people living in abject and degrading conditions. It is not the world, which is to blame for misery, but the emotional responses of humans to their troubles. The 5 steps in the book offer practical routines, which can quiet negative emotions. When you learn to control your negative emotions, you suddenly realize that nothing in the world can trouble you. You have a better ability to face problems in life, to control your environment and to accept the inevitable.

The first step to enjoying a feeling of gratitude and abundance is to know how to control your emotions. McCollough and Emmons noted that gratitude encouraged a positive cycle of reciprocal kindness among people since one act of gratitude encourages another. McCullough suggests that people can increase their sense of well-being and create positive social effects just by counting their blessings. Several exercises have been designed to increase one's experience of the emotion. Participants in such exercises showed increases in positive emotions immediately after the exercise.

One exercise is to systematically write down lists of things for which a person feels grateful each day. Another is to write a letter of gratitude or reflect on their thankfulness to someone who has obliged them. Actively experiencing the emotion has been shown to improve the outlook of people. The effect was highest for those who were more prone to feel gratitude. The obvious implication is that gratitude is more an inbuilt quality of people who are already well adjusted. Gratitude is the outcome of a healthy state of mind rather than the cause of one's sense of well being.

But, people can improve their sense of well being by frequently expressing gratitude. Fear and gratitude cannot co-exist. The pessimist feels that if anything can go wrong, it will. He anticipates trouble just around the corner. Yet his thoughts are managed by one hundred billion neurons, which ceaselessly fire thousands of times a second. Millions of people perform myriad tasks to keep him fed, clothed, and sheltered. Thousands of components in an automobile work perfectly to transport him daily to work. Modern life is a miracle of coordination, where nature and technology work together to make life possible. While the news media reports murder and mayhem, the world moves at a more sedate pace. If we believe that the world is remarkably well run, we will be better prepared to face the challenges of the few things that fail to work. We can feel grateful that all the possible things that could go wrong do not.

The expression of gratitude to the Almighty is important in Western religion. The devout feel grateful that they are showered with blessings in spite of being unworthy sinners. They feel gratitude for their calm sense of being divinely protected from harm. They accept the misfortunes and agonies of life as being divinely designed to strengthen them. But the skeptics are not so fortunate. They fail to comprehend the incessant need for misfortunes to meet a grand eternal purpose. Neither do they feel protected from random accidents and disasters. But even the hapless skeptic can also begin to feel gratitude by stilling their troubling emotions. When they begin to accept much of the surrounding misery as an irrevocable part of life and choose to enjoy the positive feelings of wonder, love, and compassion, the balance of emotions will shift in favor of gratitude. The skeptic needs to direct his gratitude.

Free from turmoil, he calmly accepts whatever is in store in life and lives mindfully, filled with wonder, love, and compassion. Life is no longer an insufferable option. Without expecting anything in return, life has given him the opportunity to live calmly and joyfully. He does not owe anyone a debt for this opportunity. Gratitude is naturally triggered when you receive an undeserved benefit. A joyful life is a priceless benefit that results from the unchanging laws of nature, which made life itself possible. Were those underlying maxims, which finally led to life, created, or did they exist forever? According to Einstein, we will never know. According to Hinduism, not even Brahma knows. But the skeptic can feel grateful that, altogether unearned and utterly gratuitously, life happened. He also knows that his gratitude will not save him from being run over by a bus because true gratitude is not felt in anticipation of future favors.

ABRAHAM THOMAS

*The Intuition Way is the first book in the world to provide the insightful 20 millisecond intuition/pattern recognition link between events, emotions and motor responses.*

# THE CRISIS OF WORTHLESSNESS

*"Self-esteem is not thinking you are better than everyone else, it's knowing that you are good enough."*

### How To Build Your Self-Esteem

Overcoming low self-esteem is a matter of learning to get rid of a painful habit. "Low self-esteem" is too mild an expression to describe its inflicted misery. Esteem is, after all, a "feeling of delighted approval and liking." People esteem ability - to fly a plane, swim the channel, or even have the capacity to deflate an arrogant shop assistant. If these things don't come easily to you, you can hardly esteem yourself in these areas. Self-esteem is also transitory - a brief enjoyment of the delight of doing something well. Any little thing can deflate your self-esteem. But low self-esteem is starkly different. It goes on and on. It is habitual and punishing self-criticism that can darken every aspect of your life. In this article, low self-esteem is defined as a habit of painful self-criticism.

Some timid children suffer from low self-esteem. They may grow up and succeed in life, since success in most jobs does not require killer instincts. Job competence alone usually takes quiet and soft-spoken people to the top. But, in spite of career success, the low self-esteem of timid people may persist. It is much worse for the less fortunate. For every success story, there are so many ordinary workers. Low self-esteem can punish them with crippling reminders that they are failures. For all these afflicted people, effective mind control is possible. A few mental and physical exercises can still prevent such habitual self-criticism. Overcoming low self-esteem will not work miracles. It will not convert quiet people into extroverts. But it will make them feel at ease in company.

The Intuition Way is a must-read for anyone who wants to understand and develop their intuition. The 5 steps in the book will calm their minds. They will feel comfortable about not being "the life of the party." They can go on to discover their hidden talents. Every individual has unique abilities. These can be exploited. Her classmates and elder brothers constantly teased Margaret. She came to feel inferior to other people. Her emotional responses to those early cat calls burned this conviction into her system. Psychologists usually regard Margaret's essential shyness as an enduring personality characteristic. She was not built to be a bully. But her low self-esteem made her forget the many instances when she did well and was praised. For her, any praise appeared false, and she constantly felt unworthy. Margaret assesses herself to be at the lowest end of the Rosenberg self-esteem scale.

She believes she is no good; that she has done nothing to be proud of; that she is useless; that she has no respect for herself; that she is a failure. Naturally, she avoids company. Her painful emotional focus blinds her to her own good qualities—the things she can do well, the times she has contributed, and those parts of her behavior that deserve respect. One reason why low self-esteem persists is that its root cause endures. Quiet people lack the skills to deal with aggressive people. Early in life, aggressive, high-self-esteem people keep winning the competition for supremacy among equals in the school yard. These pushy extroverts possess a fearsome advantage. They are born with the right tools: loud voices, aggressive natures, innate humor, or dogged persistence. They win innumerable daily battles and reach the top of the social hierarchy. Their youthful cruelty in the schoolyard inflicts the enduring emotional pain of low self-esteem on timid children.

The affected children may become rich and powerful later in life. Money or executive power may enable them to dominate subordinates. But such people lack the killer instincts needed to win in confrontations with equals. They tend to lose these "novice vs. master" battles. So, the low self-esteem mechanism keeps corroding the system. It is not usually changed with wealth and power or with positive affirmations.

It is worse for those who have not achieved career success. For them, the pain becomes more intense with the passing years. Punishing self-criticism goes on and on. Follow the methods suggested in these pages to happily overcome low self-esteem. Margaret is uncomfortable in company. Her shyness aggravates the situation. Being unable to share common jokes and comments, she feels tongue-tied and awkward in company. In reality, she cannot "will herself" to be outgoing and talkative. Consider the problem. She cannot control her complex subconscious processes.

These routines need to work with lightning speed before she can utter a word in response to a taunt. They should formulate a witty response, paraphrase it into words, select the right words from a vocabulary of thousands of words, and place them in grammatical order. Then these systems must initiate motor impulses to control the timing and tenor of her voice. All these things must happen before she responds. If Margaret is tongue-tied, it is because mechanisms over which she has no conscious control have decided to remain silent. Her reticence is not a conscious choice.

It is your mind that decides to speak. Your brain stores memories of evolutionary experiences dating back millions of years. It remembers the sights, sounds, and experiences of a lifetime. It stores the coded memories of years of habitual activities. These are astronomically large memory stores. As an example, if the DNA codes in the human body were written into 500-page books, those tomes would fill the Grand Canyon 50 times over!

Your mind recalls responses from a similarly large memory store. Over the years, high-self-esteem extroverts accumulate vast memories of successful social exchanges. Sadly, her painful schoolyard experiences form Margaret's memory store, making her motor system freeze her to avoid more pain. She cannot consciously make the system deliver witty replies or gracious words. It evaluates its own assembled memories and remains frozen. Margaret's actions are controlled by her emotions, an evolutionary control system developed by nature. Emotions compete with rationality for control in her historic triune brain, where a wise prefrontal region coexists with lower-level mammalian and reptilian systems.

It is her mammalian brain that punishes her with low self-esteem. It dominates her habitual social strategy, casting her in the role of a social outcast. Her feeble efforts to resist aggression keep failing. Her opponents are stronger or nastier in their verbal responses. She feels defeated by life. A defeated animal bows its head and creeps away, its tail between its legs. Its emotions drive it to avoid more pain. Every muscle in its body is controlled by its fear of confrontation. In Margaret's case, inner voices chide her for being a failure. The emotion eliminates all thoughts of her many successes and colors her view black.

Margaret's pain is intensified by her internal systems. Early in life, her mirror neuron network made her intensely aware of the scorn and contempt of her schoolmates. Eisenberger's research at UCLA suggests activity in the neural pain circuits when a person suffers social rejection. Her system also contains a mechanism that has a multiplier effect on distress.

For our ancestors in the jungle, being observed could mean the possibility of instant death. With civilization and culture, the danger of instant death has faded, but the shy person's system continues to initiate rising discomfort from observing eyes. It was acceptable for Margaret to be taunted by her brother at home. But those same taunts, while being observed by many in the school yard, made her want to die. Countless emotional experiences recorded such fear relationships in her amygdalae.

The amygdalae are organs in the brain that enable animals to remember and avoid pain. Lifelong "Speed dial (LTP) circuits" within them respond to the possibility of pain with fear signals. Those signals prepare the body for instant evasive action. Adrenalin increases to prepare the body for a flight or freeze response. Heartbeats increase to improve blood supply. Blood pressure rises, and breathing changes. Acidity increases in the stomach. The excretory system prepares to clear the toxin. While these actions have relevance for frantic flight in the jungle, these visceral activities merely fill Margaret with despair. Her voice circuits scold her for not doing enough to win her battles. Low self-esteem stresses both her body and mind. The neural signals that cause Margaret's low self-esteem follow logical paths. Her system recognizes images, which remotely link to her past pain, causing her despair. These signals can be stilled through purely mechanical intervention. She can learn to relax her muscles instantly and to still her visceral responses. She can learn to quiet her habitual instincts, which cause her tension in company. The 5 steps in the Intuition Wat suggest ways to still them through simple mental and physical exercises. She does not need to argue with her mind. The opinions of people about her are irrelevant.

These will keep changing. They may appreciate her in the morning and pour scorn on her in the evening. A still mind will recognize the flighty opinions of people as irrelevant. Mindfulness meditation can enable her to enjoy the little things in life. Overcoming low self-esteem, she can learn to be calmly comfortable in company. When fear is stilled, her rational brain will replace the anxiety of low self-esteem with "unconditional self-acceptance and other-acceptance." She will know that "Life is like that." In spite of all her success in life, she lacks the loud voice, aggressive outlook, innate humor, or dogged persistence that she can use to win social confrontations. She is weak in the art of social confrontation with equals or superiors with high self-esteem. Her innate nature cannot be changed. She is unlikely to return with a sharp putdown or to become the life of the party. But being comfortable, she will contribute when she clearly has something to say. Overcoming the pain of low self-esteem is a matter of accepting herself as a quiet, soft-spoken person. After all, high self-esteem is not a wonder either. It is known to often lead to frustration and violence.

Margaret will not need to fear that her tension will "spoil" a party. People usually become uncomfortable if they sense tension. They have mirror neurons, which "mirror" the behavior of others in their company. Those neurons support the generation of identical emotions within a group. Tension in one animal is conveyed quickly throughout the herd. It is a survival mechanism. So, effectively, the tensions of a self-critical person will also transmit to the group, lowering spirits all around. Instead of being a "wet blanket," when apprehension is calmly stilled, the same comfort will raise the spirit of the group. Margaret becomes a comfortable listener, leaving the extroverts to enjoy a "great party."

Many successful people have a low sense of self-esteem but do not feel incompetent. But there are many ordinary and hardworking people who suffer from the feeling of incompetence. People are basically motivated to work. Imitating their parents, ordinary people make traditional or accidental career choices. A person becomes a shop assistant because her parents have been the same. But their salaries barely meet their food, shelter, and clothing needs. They often live with the fear of losing their jobs. Cyclic labor turnover prevents them from enjoying steadfast work companionship. Such people lack a sense of fulfillment, being aware of their lowly contributions to society. In comparison with their successful relatives and friends, they feel incompetent. The answer is to do a good job or to enjoy the job.

Successful people discover and follow their areas of strength without wasting time in jobs where they are weak. Do you have an area of excellence? Are there a few things you can do better than others? The legendary management guide Peter Drucker defined excellence as the ability to easily do something that others find difficult. If you lack enthusiasm in your current job, look around for a job that can be more satisfying. Different objectives thrill different people. The signals that trigger pleasure in a person are said to be set before the age of nine. History could interest a child, who was once thrilled by the vision of an emperor's throne in a museum. Such exciting early visions can trigger abiding interests in subjects like history, art, or engineering. Discover the things that excite you.

Self-awareness can prevent you from being tied to tradition and dull habits. Very few people are blessed with the good fortune to work enthusiastically in a field they love. Millions of people are forced to work on dull routines that bore them to tears. If you do not enjoy your work but have no other option, are you going to let your dissatisfaction destroy your health and happiness? Instead of being miserable, look around and see how you can improve your performance. How does your work help your customers and the business? Study the history and practices in the field. Read about new developments. You will find that as you pay more attention to your job, it will become easier and more interesting. While you can keep looking for a better opening, you will find that the skills you learned will always help you later in life. There are situations where bullies win. You are a member of a committee where a domineering member takes over and manages affairs. Quiet people find it difficult to overcome their innate reserve and respond suitably in such situations.

Such committees, with members who do not contribute, are fated to be flawed. It is better to avoid situations where you feel you cannot contribute your mite. If you are unavoidably in such situations, calmly accept reality and do whatever is possible within your limitations. But don't let your helplessness bother you. Loudness never makes up for substance, and a calm approach will keep you ready for an opportunity, which will come one day. Happy survival is a person's greatest achievement. The famed psychiatrist Frankl writes that simple objectives helped people survive even the horrors of the Nazi concentration camps. Feelings of being a failure become irrelevant when you still your emotions and take joy in little things. Lacking high self-esteem is an advantage too, because a humble perception fits you better into society. Be glad that you are quiet and soft-spoken, without the problems of an aggressive extrovert. The Intuition Way provides a fresh and insightful look at how intuition sets your moods and attitudes. How emotions can be stilled.

When they are stilled, the background chatter vanishes. By stilling our emotions, we can free ourselves from the prejudices of our social group, the painful startle responses, the needless guilt, the glancing over our shoulders for competitors, the limitations in our lives, the put-downs and insults, the greed, the dissatisfaction, and the disappointments. As the primitive attacks of fear, resentment, and anger reduce, our intuition will trigger joy, wonder, and gratitude. We will be able to see the world with a clear and objective mind, and we will be able to enjoy the sunset because we are not feeling awful.

# THE CRISIS OF IMPATIENCE

*"Patience is not about waiting. Patience is about how you act while you are waiting."*
Joyce Meyer

### How To Inculcate Patience

Patience is a time-critical emotion that provides the energy for perseverance in a task. The emotion is positive, and it stills anger and annoyance in the face of delay or provocation. It also energizes a person to carry on. The emotion is initiated by the expectation of a reward and terminates at the expiration of the expected time period for receiving the reward. Time is critical for patience. While patience is advocated by religions as a virtue to be cultivated, it is mostly initiated and terminated by subconscious pattern recognition processes. Self-control, heredity, culture, and life experiences resolve the particular signals that initiate and switch off the patience emotion within each individual.

All religions praise the virtue of patience. The Hebrew Torah praises the patient man because he "shows much good sense, but the quick-tempered man displays folly at its height." Christianity advises believers to "be patient with all. See that no one returns evil for evil; rather, always seek what is good for each other and for all." The Quran advises Muslims to "be firm and patient, in pain and adversity, and throughout all periods of panic."

In Buddhism, patience is the ability to control one's emotions when being criticized or attacked. Both Hinduism and Buddhism advise meditation, which helps to choose a patient approach to life itself. Since devotees believe patience to be a virtue, the practice of patience brings them its own reward in the induced satisfaction of being virtuous. An expectation of the rewards of virtue grants them the patient energy to withstand trials and tribulations. Patience persists in efforts to achieve a rewarding objective. Such persistence becomes possible because a patient person is less vulnerable to the attacks of anger and annoyance in the face of setbacks. Professor Wolfram Schultz discovered that reward-oriented behavior is promoted by the release of a group of neurotransmitters by neurons in the approach or avoid system within the early reptilian part of the human brain.

These neurons detect signals in the environment that indicate the possibility of a reward within a specific time frame. The time frame is determined by the duration of effort required for past fruitful experiences. By releasing dopamine, these neurons increase neural activity in the forebrain, mainly in the prefrontal regions, where attention and analysis take place. Heightened prefrontal activity inhibits the amygdala, a major emotional center. Reduced amygdala activity causes a patient to be systemically less deterred by fear, anger, and annoyance in the face of provocation. It is not the reward but the expectation of a reward that releases dopamine. Its levels rise even if your objective is something as simple as wanting to cross the road. Increased dopamine strengthens forebrain activity, which brings clarity to objectives and makes a person feel more energetic and elated. Nature schedules the induction of such added focus and energy, timing it precisely to be sufficient to achieve desired objectives. Schultz recorded the timed release of dopamine by these neurons on detecting signals, which indicate the possibility of a reward.

Schultz noted that the release increases if the reward is greater than what is expected. It continues only for the predicted time period, when a reward can be expected. The release decreases at the end of this period. The releases stop if the rewards have become a matter of routine. Evidently, creative effort is not needed if the objective can be achieved mechanically. Thus, true patience, which overcomes obstructions creatively and without resentment, requires novelty and a systemic knowledge of the precise timing of expected rewards. An accurate judgment of the possibility of a reward, regardless of setbacks, is a prerequisite for patience. When the brain receives conflicting reports from different control nuclei in the brain, the anterior cingulate cortex (ACC) decides which brain region should decisively control the motor system. Laboratory tests reveal the function of ACC when a subject is asked to name the color of ink on a written word. While ACC is passive if the word "RED" is written in red ink, it becomes activated if "RED" is written in blue ink. ACC detects conflicts and activates those related regions, which can creatively resolve the conflict.

The knowledge of the possibility of a reward increases levels of dopamine and optimizes this judgmental system. Such activation of ACC improves the judgment of the existence of the reward. Activity in the ACC also inhibits anger and annoyance and grants energy to patience. Noted differences in levels of patience between marmosets and tamarins were not caused by the differences in the life histories, brain sizes, or social behaviors of these animals. Since the marmosets feed on gum, which takes a long time to flow from trees, those animals were prepared to wait longer. The tamarins, which feed on easily available insects, were less patient. A knowledge of the period of waiting for a reward determines the level of patience. Patience is decided by the related objective. The emotion is indicated when a person remains alert and actively engaged in life in spite of setbacks or even defeat. The objective of such a person may be peace of mind. This is the approach of Eastern religions.

A person may not persist in his efforts, accept defeat, and still be patient. The prime objective of such people is not to achieve an external goal but to meet an internal ambition.

Their goals are to accept life with equanimity. Annoyance and anger are stilled in their minds since the reward they value and receive is peace of mind. But patience in defeat can support nervous energy only if the expected reward is peace of mind. Without such energy, the emotion experienced in the face of defeat is resignation and passivity, not patience. In seeking external rewards, patience is dynamic. In his famous novel, James Clavell outlines the patience of Lord Toranaga in his efforts to conquer his last powerful rival and become the Shogun of Japan. His objective was to be alert until "one day, he will make one mistake, and then he too will be gone!" The Lord was watchful and engaged while he waited for his lethal opportunity.

Patience takes calm control of the mind, like the emotion of a fisherman sitting with a baited hook. While it is human to be occasionally overcome by negative emotions, the emotion of patience functions only during clear periods of rational thinking. A patient person perseveres without negative emotions. Those who are angry or give up are not exhibiting patience but the emotions of vexation, defeat, and despair. Patience, which struggles on despite heavy odds against success, may come from an optimistic nature. Tali Sharot scanned the brains of optimists, who sustained a positive outlook towards events (a home team winning after 10 consecutive losses). ACC monitors conflict and decides motor activity based on emotional experiences of successes and failures. The region interprets conflicting data, generating ERN (error-related negativity) for errors and ERP (positive signals) for correct answers. Tali noted that, for optimists, the ACC appeared to be more active.

Their positive expectations of a reward endured longer. Just as motor impulses continue firing to contract muscles until the target is achieved, dopamine release continues longer for optimists, powering them to persist longer. Though their judgments may be biased, they are likely to be more patient in their efforts. Patience is triggered by subconscious signals of expected rewards. The reward may be as simple as reaching a counter while standing in a queue. The governing criterion is the internally expected timing of the reward. The energy and interest triggered by patience vanish when that expected period of waiting is over. For those prone to impatience, the simple remedy may be to accept the possibility of a longer wait or even that the counter will close before it is reached.

The instinctive time-evaluation component of patience exists in humans and animals. Normally, both tend to choose quick, short-term rewards over larger, longer-term rewards. Marmosets were found to be more patient than the tamarins. Patience tests on these animal species, giving them the option to pick a lesser reward immediately or wait longer for a more substantial reward revealed that the marmosets waited significantly longer than the tamarins.

Patience comes from a realistic assessment of the time it takes to achieve a reward. Like marmosets, a willingness to wait helps in all aspects of life. When such an objective is expressed consciously, those waiting periods at traffic lights or in queues can become periods when the mind becomes relaxed and refreshed. When the reward is seen as peace of mind, such periods will also fill the mind with energy.

CHAPTER 18

# THE CRISIS OF SEVERE GUILT

*"Guilt is a useless emotion. It's never enough to make us change our behavior, and it only serves to make us feel worse." - Wayne Dyer*

### How To Live With The Pain Of Guilt

Ann surely needs help dealing with severe guilt. A few years ago, she swung out onto the outer lane to overtake a slow-moving van and collided head-on with an oncoming truck. Her husband was killed on the spot, and her son was paralyzed from the waist down. Years later, her sense of guilt continues to blame her cruelly for her fatal error of judgment.

A feeble and pained voice within her keeps rejoining with the truth—that it was just a momentary mistake that could have happened to anyone.

It was just one thoughtless but awful mistake. Each time Ann opens her front door and feels the emptiness, each time she glimpses her child in the wheelchair, the painful voice returns, hurting her with its relentless logic. Her stern guilt and despair poison her career and the upbringing of her son, transforming her life into a living nightmare. In dealing with severe guilt, Ann needs to get her shattered life back on an even keel. She needs to realize that she can learn to control the evolutionary neural mechanisms that torture her. She can calmly come to terms with her guilt, which is merely a social emotion, triggered by her nervous system, to control her behavior.

As Ann's nervous system evolved over millions of years, nature developed increasingly complex control patterns to enable survival. The early reptilian brains responded to smells, fear, and anger. Smells determined whether an object could be approached or avoided. Fear and anger decided whether the animal should retreat or attack. Those control decisions supported individual survival. Further evolution led to the mammalian brain, where social emotions controlled herd behavior. Guilt and shame punished any selfish behavior that broke the moral code of the group. The emotions triggered drives, which opposed unsocial actions and compelled members to act for the group's benefit. Pain at the prospect of social rejection became wired into the system.

Eisenberger's research at UCLA confirms activity in the neural pain circuits when a person suffers social rejection. A person suffers pain when damaged skin cells cause nociceptors (pain nerve cells) to fire. Such pain processing is reported to have two parallel channels. The first causes the sensation of pain, and the second causes the feeling of being "hurt." The "hurt" experience is more disagreeable than the pain sensation. Fear compels an animal to escape from or avoid a source of pain.

To enable animals to remember and avoid pain, "speed dial circuits" persist over the years in the amygdala, the organ associated with fear. Those circuits trigger distress when they recognize any pattern remotely linked to the original source of pain. Eisenberger suggests that the same circuits are activated in the case of guilt. Ann cannot run away from her misjudgment. So, the drive triggers internal voice circuits, accusing her of her guilt upon recognition of any associated pattern. When dealing with severe guilt, Ann needs to understand that pattern recognition and speed dial circuits are also the reasons for her punishment.

Evolutionary development led to the common-sense regions of the prefrontal human brain. Scientists are surprised that a bunch of nerve cells can have a conscience. But they acknowledge the vast extent of knowledge contained in the DNA molecule in each living cell in the human body. If inscribed into 500-page books, the programmed DNA codes in the human body would fill the Grand Canyon 50 times over with those books! Nerve cells contain similar masses of code in their combinatorial codes.

The prefrontal cortex contains the accumulated wisdom of millions of years and the memories of a lifetime of sensory and emotional experiences. That brain has the wisdom to know what is right and wrong in the vast turmoil of human relations and social responsibilities. When her common sense tells her that she made a wrong decision that caused grievous harm, Her common sense is right. That judgment of her common sense triggers her overactive guilt and pain circuits. But her common sense will also tell her that that mistake could have been made by anyone. That she should accept her error and move on. In dealing with deep grief, Ann should understand that the speed dial circuits always enhance her pain and still the small inner voice of her common sense.

Ann can never hope to argue with her feelings of guilt and win. In reality, her actions were wrong. But she can switch off her guilt circuit. She can use a foible of the nervous system: when the attention of the mind is directed to the onset of an emotion, the emotion is instantly stilled. The attention of the mind is the attention of the prefrontal regions.

Normally, when an emotion takes over, her prefrontal region is only an observer who feels the pain. But if you consciously begin to observe your mind, Your common sense will take over. It will be possible to see the onset of thoughts triggered by lower-level animal emotions in the mammalian part of the triune human brain. Your common sense will become able to identify the sharp, accusing voices of guilt and still them through mere observation. It is similar to the age-old advice to count up to ten before you speak harshly. Shift the attention of your mind, and anger will disappear. Ann should know that self-awareness will not come overnight. In dealing with severe grief, it will require observation over a period of time for her to become familiar with her troubling thoughts, just as she knows her annoying acquaintances.

The Buddhists discovered the path of self-awareness and mindfulness meditation, which grants control of your mind to your common sense. It is a powerful investigative intelligence that "sees the flower as being neither beautiful nor ugly." According to unemotional common sense, it is just a flower. The mind-control tips on this website suggest a few mental and physical exercises to put your common sense in charge. Those exercises can still your animal instincts with their speed dial circuits, which respond to every hint and shake you around like a puppet on a string.

In time, the practice of those routines will transport your mind to calm, neutral territory. In successfully dealing with severe guilt, these practices can enable Ann to live sensibly with her disastrous mistake. With its immense inherent wisdom, her common sense knows it was a mistake. It also knows of the fallibility of humans and of the need to move on beyond disaster. Ann will view the problems ahead and the mistakes of the past as "like birds in the sky." They are there, but they do not matter.

The love emotion activates the affiliation network, which can still feel the pain of guilt. Self-compassion training grants sufficient control of the mind to enable a practitioner to consciously switch on the network. The initiation creates a powerfully positive attitude. A loving acceptance of the pain of the self takes place. The guilty person will feel compassion for the poor, suffering self, which will act to reduce the pain of guilt.

A stable social life requires ways to deal with conflicts and events in which people inadvertently (or even purposefully) harm others. If a person harms someone, guilt causes him to express regret and sorrow, which is likely to be forgiven. In this way, the chances of retaliation are reduced, and the community fares better. A person who feels no guilt is likely to harm others and be destroyed, in the end, by society. At one time or another, everyone makes a mistake, commits an error of judgment, or says or does something wrong.

Self-awareness can make each person listen to the voice of conscience. Remember that it is an immensely wise intelligence that triggers your feeling of guilt. Act to remedy the situation. Apologize to the person and express your sorrow at your error. Avoid repeating the behavior. Each such incident will improve your sensitivity to people and prevent the serious deterioration of your personal relationships. You may not be dealing with severe guilt. But you can use guilt as your wise guide and counselor to grow, learn, and mature.

Our minds contain a neural subsystem that senses the feelings of others and makes us feel the same emotions. These neurons are called mirror neurons. This system makes us feel the sufferings of others and triggers the compassion emotion. The emotion triggers a drive to make us act to mitigate the suffering. When we are unable to help, feelings of guilt are triggered.

People who are sensitive to these feelings are likely to be cooperative and altruistic. But they are also more likely to suffer from anxiety and depression. Such suffering is intensified by the conviction of their common sense that it is their duty to help. Peace of mind can come only when RI systematically evaluates all options and makes a competent value judgment for the circumstances surrounding each such periodic pang of guilt that overtakes them. Each person has to make a choice about the extent of altruistic behavior that can be afforded in the turmoil of everyday life.

One of the five steps in the Intuition Way is to become self-aware. Self-awareness will make you sensitive to any discomfort over some event during the day. To follow this plan, you can write down all your thoughts about this issue the way you would write a shopping list. Your mind has the capacity to search through its vast memories to bring you all the thoughts surrounding this concern. The plan offers a way to organize these thoughts and enable your common sense to understand your concern.You may not have the time or resources to improve a situation.

- You may have chosen a career instead of staying at home.
- You may not be as good as someone else at dealing with the problem.
- You may not achieve the perfection in your work that you expect of yourself.
- You may have felt anger toward someone you care for.

- Circumstances may have forced you to accept help.
- Changing your behavior may cause you too much distress.
- You may not be able to change a mistake from the past.
- You may have acted wrongly with the only information available to you.
- The problem could have occurred regardless of all your efforts.

Writing it down will bring out the many conflicting views within your mind. The plan enables you to make your choices. Knowing the rationale behind your choice will prevent this sense of guilt from coming up again. You will not feel trapped. Your common sense will have understood and made its choices. Your behavior will slowly be modified to meet your decision. When dealing with severe guilt, it is also important to tone down such feelings, which may run in your subconscious.

Your common sense knows whether you smoke or eat too much. It knows that regular exercise is good for you. You feel guilt when you act against the judgment of your common sense. You may have always intended to break your bad habits or begin good ones. Yet, when you get down to it, you lack the willpower. Actually, you fail in this conflict between your common sense and your animal instincts because emotions control your life. Your nervous system always shifts to your most powerful emotion. When hunger pangs, a need for a smoke, or sheer tiredness overcome you, you will give in to one of these habitual weaknesses.

But self-awareness can still be an emotion. If you become

conscious of the emotion, it will be stilled. Do not argue with emotion. When you are about to indulge yourself, think, "What do I feel?" instead of thinking, "I should not do this." Recognition of the physical symptoms of the emotion, which misdirect you, will kill the emotion. Your guilt is continually warning you. Use self-awareness to take control of your life. These practices will always assist you, even as you work on dealing with severe guilt.

*The Intuition Way is the first book in the world to provide the insightful 20 millisecond intuition/pattern recognition link between events, emotions and motor responses.*

# THE CRISIS OF DISAPPOINTMENT

*"Don't let disappointment stop you from trying again."*
Joyce Meyer

**Understand The Emotional Triggers That Punish You**

Your expectations of a happy outcome failed to emerge. Surely, you deserved the positive outcome. What happened was surprising and could not be controlled through your personal actions. You even suspect that you will not get, or ever achieve, what you genuinely want. What you feel is not a sense of regret about your own actions but distress, tinged with sadness or anger, over the outcome. You wish to escape this overwhelming sense of helpless gloom. Take heart. There are actions you can take to calmly accept the mishap, still the distress, and move on.

The stressful emotions you feel are instinctive and impulsive reactions to a letdown. You can overcome the agitation when your mind shifts away from its emotional viewpoint. A changed outlook will banish the cycling "what might have been" images in your mind and still the nagging sense of sadness. Disappointment is a frequent and negative emotion. It provides a graded response. The greater the anticipation, the greater the disappointment. The emotion can lead to depression. You must act to replace disappointment with creative excitement and joy by understanding and overcoming the emotional triggers of turmoil in your mind. Follow these steps to reach a sense of creative calm. Then you will make a practical plan to move on.

Nature uses disappointment to teach you how to make crucial decisions when faced with uncertainty. It is a powerful emotion that calibrates actual outcomes against your expectations. Damasio's Somatic Marker Hypothesis suggests that emotional calibration is crucial to complex decision-making. Life throws you many conflicting options. According to the scientist Frijda, emotions, their bodily effects, and the desire to enjoy or avoid similar experiences in the future determine your choices. Your mind is constantly recording your significant experiences with a calibrated range of emotions.

Such finely differentiated grades of experienced emotions

enable you to make wise choices. Stronger emotions prevail over weaker ones. Your mind makes those subtle choices that empower rational thinking, including reward anticipation and decision-making. Your distress marks the event that proved that your judgment has been seriously wrong. You feel really bad. But the event has made you wiser. But the effect of the emotion is to shift the goals of your mind away from a search for opportunities to the fearful avoidance of problems. This troubling effect is caused by the lateral habenula (LHb), a pea-sized bundle of nerves in your brain. You should not be affected by a faulty program in your nervous system.

Since life is full of uncertainty, LHb adjusts your goals by keeping track of your information-prediction and reward-prediction errors. If your expectation of increased sales did not materialize, you made an informational prediction error. If your expectation of a raise did not materialize, you made a reward prediction error. Since you failed to predict such mishaps, LHb assumes that you have false expectations of life. LHb weighs your setbacks (without counting your blessings) to conclude that your activities will lead relentlessly into disaster. It sets off a series of neural actions to motivate you to retire from all activity. To overcome your disappointment, you must understand that it is your LHb that colors your world black. The organ creates a bias in your mind by triggering neurotransmitters, which cause a loss of energy in the system.

The studies of Schimmack on the frequency and intensity of emotions in real-life events found that disappointment is one of the most frequent and negative of such emotions. It provides a graded response. The greater the anticipation, the greater the disappointment. According to Steven Shabel, disappointment is signaled by the release of the neurotransmitter glutamate by LHb. When more glutamate is released, the more intense the disappointment signals are, which spread in the system. Disappointment stimulates the parasympathetic nervous system. The chemical responses lead to melancholy, inertia, and a feeling of hopelessness. The heightened sense of dismay leads to increased expectations of future letdowns.

The setback envelops you in feelings of helplessness. You lose interest in your daily routines. There is a loss of energy and self-criticism. Your appetite and sleep are affected. Your problems look bigger, and you worry about problems that could happen. You feel scared without any specific or direct threat. You become more prone to anger and irritability. Your actions become less well-considered and more impulsive. This continuing emotional roller coaster can lead to heart disease, digestive disorders, and a depressed immune system. All this is triggered by a changed balance of chemicals in the habenula.

You have no awareness of the intuitive process that activated LHb and enabled your animal instincts to take over. Reduced dopamine availability in the forebrain has lessened your energy. Intuition has inhibited the memories of lilting songs and bright mornings to morbidly convince you that your situation is hopeless. It is not. A simple mental exercise can stop this whole knee-jerk process in its tracks.

Your common sense will take control and set free memories of sunshine and laughter. All you need is a little practice in self-awareness. Learn to become aware when emotional turmoil begins within you. Self awareness is the key theme in the meditation practiced for centuries by the Buddhists. They recommended "staring back" at your thoughts.

Matthieu Ricard, a respected Buddhist monk, said: "One may wonder what people do in retreats, sitting for eight hours a day. They familiarize themselves with a new way of dealing with the arising of thoughts." "When you start getting used to recognizing thoughts as they arise, it is like rapidly spotting someone you know in a crowd. When a powerful thought or anger arises, you recognize it. That helps you avoid being overwhelmed by this thought." Self-awareness enables you to recognize your depression as just a transitory mood.

The vicious cycles of thoughts that cause you anguish can be stilled through self-awareness. Recognize the turmoil in your mind. The shattered images of your expectations of a bright future cause endless reruns of "what might have been" images in your mind. Each image of missed opportunities increases the discharge of glutamate by LHb. Just awareness that your mind is in turmoil leads you to the next thought. What can you do about it? You can take a series of mental steps to still the anguish.

The first thing to do is face up to the worst impact of your disappointing outcome. Can you live with it? Think of the repercussions. You will have to admit that the earth will keep spinning and the sun will rise again. Life will still go on. Facing up to your letdown is a purifying exercise. The flailing in a cage feeling stops. Directly facing the consequences of the mishap will stop the "might have been" reruns. The turmoil remains, but you recognize your disappointment not as an overwhelming world view but as a sad event in your life. What action can you take now?

Your earlier expectations had filled you with hope and excitement. After the letdown, you face a bleak future. Look around and evaluate your expectations. Hindsight grants you a better view of the real world. Your mind will store this outcome and bring it up the next time you face an uncertain choice. What was the possibility that you ignored? Was that a freak event or a reasonable likelihood? Plan your future course of action in light of this new knowledge.

If you expected to win a million in a lottery, one hundred thousand will be a disappointment. If you have experienced intense disappointment before, it may be an indication that your expectations are too high. Lowering your targets will not kill your dreams. You only become more practical. Consciously lower your expectations in the future to achieve a more balanced emotional life. Evaluate the reasons for the letdown and see if you can improve the outcome with more resources or better planning. Detach yourself from a losing cause.

Disappointment is nature's way of jolting you into reality. But don't let disappointment breed pessimism. It is a feeling that envelops you in gloom. The intuitive process acts globally. It manipulates all your memories. It darkens your horizons by preventing you from recalling all your past successes. It prevents you from fighting back.

Decision analysts operate on the assumption that individuals will try to avoid the potential for disappointment and make decisions that are less likely to lead to the experience of it. When feeling disappointed, a person is more likely to sell at a loss. Give yourself time to come out of the low mood. Make your important decisions only after the sense of hopelessness leaves you.

A depressed outlook is the result of reduced forebrain activity. Shift the focus of your mind to simple tasks that you enjoy. Play computer games, polish silver, or walk in the park. Any activity that interests you The human mind operates at its highest level when it anticipates a reward. Professor Wolfram Schultz discovered that reward-oriented behavior is promoted by the release of a group of neurotransmitters by neurons in the early reptilian part of the human brain.

These neurons detect signals in the environment that indicate the possibility of a reward within a specific time frame. By releasing dopamine, these neurons increase neural activity in the forebrain. Dopamine increases alertness, provides clarity for immediate objectives, and makes a person feel more energetic and elated. Schultz noted that the release continues only for the predicted time period, when a reward can be expected. The release decreases at the end of this period. The releases stop if the rewards have become a matter of routine.

Your work needs some novelty to sustain interest. The solution to each new problem, however simple, provides a reward. Studies indicate that energy does not require engagement in creative or artistic tasks. It is experienced even in tasks such as analyzing data or filling out income tax returns. Swift answers the challenges of a job grant with energy. As you continue your task, you will come out of your mood of hopelessness.

The future that you looked forward to has vanished. The human mind needs a purpose to become strong and vibrant. The famed psychiatrist Frankl suggested that, even when life looked hopeless, a purpose was absolutely needed for survival. Having encountered the horrors of the Nazi concentration camps, he learned that people could survive torture and beatings if they had a purpose in life. But these were not large purposes. The hope of meeting a son after the war was a purpose. Even a decision to harden oneself against suffering was sufficient. After the war, Frankl established a major field in psychiatry, assisting thousands of suicidal patients around the world to recover by discovering an acceptable purpose in life. After your disappointment, you too need to find an acceptable purpose. Enjoy the feeling that you are better prepared to meet the uncertainties of life. After all, trying to avoid disappointment will make you overly cautious.

Treat this experience as a footnote to avoid distress if similar things happen again. Change your goals to overcome your errors. Can you set an easier goal? Can you reach your goal by attempting less ambitious steps? Can you get helpful advice? Can you follow the steps of those who succeeded? In the end, disappointment improves your ability to predict the future. Benefit from the powerful lesson granted to you by nature.

ABRAHAM THOMAS

*The Intuition Way is the first book in the world to provide the insightful 20 millisecond intuition/pattern recognition link between events, emotions and motor responses.*

CHAPTER 20

# FREE WILL WITHIN LIMITS

*"Free will is a complex issue, but it is clear that
we have some degree of freedom.
We are not just puppets of our genes
or our environment. We can make choices,
and those choices matter." - Massimo Pigliucci*

The denial of the existence of a free will attacks the fundamental concept of human moral responsibility. If actions are not freely chosen, there can be no judgments of praise, guilt, or sin. If all decisions of the mind are predetermined, advice, persuasion, deliberation and prohibition are meaningless. Much of scientific research does reveal the existence of deterministic controls over the choices of the mind. Consider the evidence.

When you begin to talk, your nervous system has already assigned control of your speech to a feeling. It has articulated an idea around the emotion, chosen apt words, arranged them in lexical and grammatical order and adjusted the pitch of your voice. You have no conscious inkling of what words you will use. If you do not even know what words you are going to use the next moment, you are evidently not in control. That can be interpreted as the lack of a free will. But, imagine that, while nature has set safety limits on your behavior, it empowers you with vast wisdom to discover new and creative solutions to the problems you face. Creativity within limits is true freedom.

Determinists hold that everything, including our choices, are the necessary results of a sequence of causes. Chrysippus said "Everything that happens is followed by something else which depends on it by causal necessity. Likewise, everything that happens is preceded by something with which it is causally connected. For nothing exists or has come into being in the cosmos without a cause. The universe will be disrupted and disintegrate into pieces and cease to be a unity functioning as a single system, if any uncaused movement is introduced into it."

Causal determinists propose the Laplace's demon thought experiment. Imagine an entity, which knows all the laws of nature and all past and present facts. Such an entity will theoretically predict exactly how you will act. Logical determinists suggest that since a future event is either true, or false, your action tomorrow can only be the action, which is one of two possible true predictions today. For theological determinists, an omnipotent entity has decided and knows your action tomorrow. In all three cases, a free will is impossible. But, there are compatibilists, who believe that a free will can coexist with determinism.

Religions generally support the concept of a free will, while believing in an omnipotent creator. The primary approach of Christian belief makes free choice logically impossible. But, the philosopher Kierkegaard suggested that divine omnipotence cannot be separated from divine goodness. A good God could create beings with true freedom over God, because "the greatest good ... which can be done for a being, greater than anything else that one can do for it, is to be truly free."

According to Islamic doctrine free will is the main factor for man's accountability. All actions taken by man's free will are said to be counted on the Day of Judgment, because they are his own and not God's. The concept of karma in Hinduism is generally linked to the determination of a person's destiny in future lives.

For Buddhism, the idea that a person has complete freedom of choice is foolish, because it denies the reality of one's physical needs and circumstances. Equally incorrect is the idea that we have no choice in life or that our lives are predetermined. To deny freedom would be to undermine the efforts of Buddhists to make moral progress, freely choosing compassionate action.

According to Sam Harris, the thoughts and intentions of people emerge from causes of which they are unaware. They exert no conscious control over them. Every choice they make is made as a result of preceding causes and is therefore not really a choice at all. Essentially biochemical puppets, humans lack a free will. Effects have followed causes from the beginning of time. Science suggests that a ten billion degree sea of particles existed just one second after the big bang. The patterns of their interactions were precisely ordered and stable across billions of years. When life did not exist, there was just a relentless chain of mindless causes and effects. Such determinism pointed finally to eternal darkness.

Determinism means causal determinism. But, imagine the possibility of choice determinism, which has been valid since the beginning of life. In a living environment, purposive choices move relentlessly towards intended goals. This axiom also has been validated by the abundance of life. Consider the flagellum, present in virtually all living cells. It is driven by proton motive force, with a rotor, which rotates at up to 1,00,000 rpm. With a clutch and a brake, it can reverse directions in a 1/4 turn. This microscopic water cooled engine powers the purposeful movement of living cells. An astonishing collection of such molecules proved that choice determinism could achieve an incredible variety of goals.

Choice determinism was the driving force of life. Instead of a cause-effect response, a living thing had many available options for responses. With purposeful choice, an event that follows one choice out of many moves towards the intended outcome. Nature made that choice using knowledge. Nature created intelligent systems, which store memories of trillions of causes and effects. Each of those intelligent entities selects the most appropriate of all its possible choices to meet its goal. You are such a choice deterministic system, with a complex array of supporting intelligences. They include the raw drives of a reptilian brain, the social restrictions of a mammalian brain, the rational common sense of the prefrontal regions (PFR) and consciousness, a conscious intelligence.

Determinism is not the problem if, sometimes, you are limited to one choice among many. $2 + 2 = 4$. If you face a deadly predator, run away. Even a consequentialist approach to criminal justice suggests that, at the deepest levels, consequences can control your decisions. The wisdom of your mind tries to limit you to those logical choices. A slew of such options switch in to assist you without your request.

Emotions are an example. Paul Eckman said "We become aware a quarter, or half second after the emotion begins. I do not choose to have an emotion, to become afraid, or to become angry. I am suddenly angry. I can usually figure out later what someone did that caused the emotion." Knee jerk responses are not appropriate expressions of free will. But, those emotional supporting systems are not compelling you to decide. Nature has given you the power to control emotions. If you take the time and effort, you can shut down the knee-jerk mechanisms and have a truly free will.

People tend to confuse nature's suggestions with compulsions. Science has managed to capture the mechanisms at the critical point where nerve impulses enter conscious awareness. Objects or events in the real world have many attributes, including color, shape, distance, velocity, smell, sound and feel. A PET study by Hadjikhani revealed the involvement of the claustrum in cross-model matching, in tasks that require the simultaneous evaluation of information from more than one sensory domain.

Without this structure, the subject may still be able to respond to simple, isolated or to highly familiar stimuli, but not to complex or unfamiliar ones. The claustrum perceives objects and events in an integrated manner and not as isolated attributes. This region, your conscious intelligence, routinely lets a bewildering array of fears and resentments to enter your consciousness. The claustrum may compel you to choose, if you are gullible.

Benjamin Libet discoverd that consciousness is just a belated observer of the activities of your mind. He studied subjects who voluntarily pressed a button, while noting the position of a dot on a computer screen, which shifted its position every 43 milliseconds. The noted moment of depressing the button was the moment of conscious awareness; the exact instant the subject thought the button was pressed. Each time, Libet had also timed the beginning of motor neuron activity in the brains of his subjects. He discovered that awareness occurred 350 milliseconds AFTER the beginning of motor activity. When you strike out in anger, the system has already taken charge. You are not consciously making your decisions.

Try this thought experiment. Can your will raise your hand? Yes, when you are sitting quietly in your room. But, suppose you are in an elevator with other passengers. Then, it is improper for you to raise your arms. If you consciously will this action in that situation, it will not happen. The wise system has over ruled your conscious will, because the action is not appropriate. The exercise of your will is subject to clear restrictions. Your conscious will can initiate an action only if it is worthwhile, appropriate, safe and practical. In an airliner, you will not be permitted to take unsafe actions that will crash the machine, when its autopilot is on. When you raised your hand in your room, your will controlled the system. Subject to fail safe systems, you are the pilot, the entity in charge of your nervous system.

Manufacturing lines apply automated decision making. A machine identifies a component, picks it up from a conveyor and drops it into an appropriate bin. The machine is designed to make choices and act, when switched on. Imagine that free will is also an automatic mechanism which triggers the next highest priority activity of the system, while the system is awake. The brain is designed to recognize situations, identify strategies, and act decisively. Decision making is at the core of the system. Human consciousness has a delayed view of the cause and the effect. Libet's experiments showed that the conscious view occurred a few hundred milliseconds after the the actual event.

While just an observer, consciousness has a three dimensional view of the world, appears to make decisions and experiences life. The brain recognizes that observer as "I." It positions the observer at the focal point of vision - behind our eyes, just below the top of our heads. Proprioceptors confirm the location of "I" with a "feel" for the position of our arms and legs. To the brain, "I" is a physical presence, with an uncanny perception of the world. A ghost in the machine. But, an independent "I" in the brain is as real as an "I" in a thermostat. "I" is a confused mental construct. The brain is the real "I."

The philosopher Rudolf Steiner suggested that true freedom of action existed only "when conscious awareness was integrated with moral imagination in making decisions." The goal of the moral person is to choose a course of action without external coercion in accordance with his ideals or moral outlook. Life introduced the phenomenon of purposeful choice into the cause and effect chain. The choice determinism of life achieves goals. The goal of the moral person is to decide independently to act with a moral conscience. Moral choices are the right choices. Such choices are impossible if your action is impractical, irrational, or ruled by negative emotions. The choice determinism of moral purpose is that its actions move relentlessly towards moral results. PFR decisions are free, practical and unemotional. But, such free will is also deterministic. The right choice is your only available choice.

Nature has endowed you with the most powerful intelligence in the known universe. It has many components. Several of them will prevent you from acting suicidally. One (your consciousness) makes you aware of your current state of mind. Many others (your emotional drives) use the experience of millions of years to recommend that you fight, or flee. Still another, (your PFR) takes the experiences of millions of years and those of a lifetime to offer you the best possible options. When your PFR makes decisions, your will is free and you will be judged guilty or be praised for your actions. You are open to advice, persuasion, deliberation and prohibition by society. When your PFR is in control, you are not a puppet driven by the system. You have the power to enable the component you will use. The wisdom of your mind makes the right choice considering all the knowledge available to it. It is a totally logical pattern recognition process.

Centuries ago, the Buddhists had discovered that emotions could be stilled. Self awareness was the key to quieting emotions and empowering the PFR. While the beneficial results of self awareness are soothing, the changes in your viewpoints happen slowly. You have to keep exploring the strange thought patterns, which float up into your consciousness. As you scrutinize them, your system grasps its own irrationalities and begins to rewrite miles of code. The process sets you free. You occupy a simple observation mode, which effortlessly stills the attacks of fear, resentment or anger. Then, your consciousness will confirm to you that you are truly free. A truly free intelligence does live within your mind. But you have to empower it.

CHAPTER 21

# BE AN OPTIMIST

*"The pessimist sees the difficulty
in every opportunity; the optimist sees
the opportunity in every difficulty."*
Winston Churchill

If you are a pessimist, you see the world to be as bad as it can possibly be. It is a negative view of life, which is harmful to your health. So, develop a new "explanatory style" to change your gloomy view into a vision of a bright and cheerful world.

That view needs an understanding that your happiness comes from within you and that events follow a universal pattern with a stable order. Pessimism is based on an internal conviction that you have no control over events, which occur erratically, without any universally applicable pattern.

A change in your convictions will rewire the neural circuits, which support that view. Your mind and its responses will improve. Your habitual patterns of thought will become brighter.

Both optimism and pessimism originate from subconscious pattern recognition. Those attitudes may partially be inherited, but are acquired largely through experiences in life. Extensive research on groups of optimists and pessimists show mixed results. Among those suffering from rheumatoid arthritis, or asthma, optimists were not more likely than pessimists to report pain alleviation, or to be psychologically better adjusted. But, optimists emerge from difficult circumstances with less distress than do pessimists.

Optimism has links to good health, including preventative health. An optimist is less likely to experience illness. Optimism reduces the severity and duration of an illness and reduces the possibilities of relapses. Sadly, while it is nice to be an optimist, the attitude is subconscious and a pessimist cannot just "will" himself to be an optimist. A change requires your inner wisdom to absorb a few important insights.

A pessimistic interpretation of an event is not your conscious choice. Your mind senses patterns and acts, before you know it. The famous experiments of Benjamin Libet demonstrated your essential helplessness. He showed that, even when you voluntarily press a button, your motor systems begin to act 350 milliseconds BEFORE you think you have pressed it. Subconscious processes make your decisions, way ahead of your conscious awareness.

Within the instant in which your eyes perceive a group of black and white pixels on this page, your mind interprets them as a set of characters forming a word and locates its meaning. As you read, myriad entities evaluate vast memories, compare your experiences, recall childhood images, and pass judgment on the validity of this paragraph. You merely become aware of the final conclusion. If you wish to change from pessimism to optimism, your vast subconscious mind has to become convinced that optimism is both justified and desirable.

Pessimists challenge a belief in the potential for endless progress as well as the general religious view that "this is the best of all possible worlds." Arthur Schopenhauer speaks for pessimism. According to him, human beings are motivated by hunger, sexuality, the need to care for children and the need for personal security and shelter. Driven by these needs, the selfish instincts of mankind generally overcome its rationality. This creates endless and pointless conflicts for earth's limited resources, which will continue till the extinction of the human race. For Schopenhauer, life presently exists with great difficulty. If things had been worse, the human race would not have existed. He reasons that, since a worse world could not exist, we live in the worst of all possible worlds.

Murphy's Law "If anything can go wrong, it will" is the refrain of the pessimists. Pessimists focus on the things that can go wrong. But, billions of things do not go wrong. Myriad neurons in your nervous system, the complex circuits of your monitor and computer, the worldwide circuits of the internet, power stations, distribution systems, all do not go wrong for you to be able to read these lines. The baser instincts of humanity did not prevent the progress of human civilization from famine and disease to the world of science and medicine. But, then,

Hitler's gas chambers are also recent history. So, regardless of whether many, or a few things do go wrong, the world goes on. Optimism and pessimism are merely viewpoints. An optimist feels gratitude for the trillions of things that do not go wrong, while a pessimist moans over the things, which can and do go wrong. Optimism (and happiness) come from the convictions of your inner wisdom.

Pessimism is merely a habitual thought pattern. It appears to be reasonable as the world encounters Alvin Toffler's Future Shock – the shattering stress and disorientation triggered by "too much change happening in too short a time." Civilization seems to be sinking into moral decay, where the cherished values of Christian/Greek/Hindu philosophy appear abandoned. Government encroachments into private lives appear to head into the "thought police" and "doublethink" narrated by George Orwell in his novel *Nineteen Eighty-Four*. But, even for a pessimist, these are extreme views. But they are considered judgments.

Your judgments of the outcome of events is made by the anterior cingulate cortex (ACC). The organ evaluates the history of your successes and failures to make its decisions. ACC has strong links to the amygdala, the organ, which triggers fear and anger in the nervous system. Their oversensitive circuits trigger negative emotions, which influence ACC judgments.

The pain of a a failure, or a loss triggers persistent LTP circuits in the amygdala, causing it to become sensitive over a lifetime to threatening signals. Impulses from the organ to the brainstem trigger (typically jumpy) avoidance behaviors. They activate the sympathetic nervous system, raising blood pressure and heart beats. These impulses sent to the facial nerves generate expressions of anger, fear, or disgust. Those impulses release neurochemicals, which increase the intensity of fight, flight or freeze responses. Normally, the sensory inputs, which imply threats would only generate a momentary response from the system. But, LTP builds up during a crisis in life. Later, it generates persisting control impulses, which converts a momentary response into persisting distress.

LTP circuits in the amygdala influence ACC causing the negative thought patterns of the pessimist. ACC normally builds on current experience of successes and failures to frame its decisions. It decides whether a person will be optimistic or pessimistic about the outcomes of his efforts in life. Those judgments are dictated by the emotional LTP inputs from the amygdala of past failures. If ACC is dominated by memories of failure, you will be a pessimist. But, if you can build up memories of successes in the amygdala by changing its viewpoint and recalling past successes, ACC can decide to make you an optimist.

Pessimists should reexamine their expectations from life. A person's goals decide whether good, or bad things happen. Optimists expect to meet their goals and pessimists expect to fail. The pessimist cannot meet his goals, because his goals have unreasonable expectations. Pessimists expect to discover a larger meaning for their life. They expect a benevolent outcome for life in the long march of history. They expect human beings to behave with nobility and altruism. They expect that fate will not deliver nasty surprises. The gloom of the pessimists rests on their inner conviction that such expectations will not be met. Pessimists need to understand that finding cosmic meaning, the arrival of utopia, the operation of an altruistic world, or the expectation of a benign fate are all irrational goals in life.

Do you worry about the meaning of your life? The deeply religious believe that their lives meet a divine purpose. But, the pessimistic skeptic will never discover a cosmic meaning for his life. Individual contributions to history have always been irrelevant. The vast empires, grand civilizations and the struggles of untold generations have vanished into the misty past without a trace. Like a grain of sand in the desert, earth circles one among billions of stars in the Milky Way Galaxy - one lone galaxy, among billions of such galaxies. In the vastness of cosmos, the pessimist vainly searches for the meaning of his life. Without such worries, the optimist discovers satisfactions within the boundless spaces of his own mind. His joy comes from his awesome capacity to grasp the immensity of space and the vast depths of history. The true optimist is happy, living in his own mind.

Like a glass, which can be both half full and half empty, both pessimism and optimism are justifiable. It is only that the optimist lives in a happier world. If the pessimist wishes to relocate, he has to see his one sided reasoning. The meaning of his life is irrelevant. Only self awareness can educate the pessimist of his habitual focus on gloom and doom. He has to become aware of the rise of negative thoughts. The immense capacity of his mind should focus on discovering the brighter side of his world.

Improved education, health and prosperity are spreading to billions of people. Each day brings amazing products and services to improve the quality of human lives. The pessimist should consciously search for hopeful events and headlines. Actively discover silver linings around dark clouds. While initially difficult, the pessimist will become skilled with practice. New LTP "speed dial circuits" will grow in his mind. Soon, he will begin to see real change within. His creativity will grow and the world will look brighter. Actually, the world will not have changed. But the vast internal worlds within the pessimist will have taken a brighter hue.

Pessimism often follows a serious disappointment in life, like the loss of a loved one, or a career setback. Since such events occur unexpectedly, usually just following a happy view of the world, pessimists fear that optimism could be a harbinger of disaster. Imagining an optimistic solution to their problems fills them with disquiet. But, optimism does not presage trouble. It favors a happier outcome. An expectation of victory triggers more successful strategies than a fear of defeat. An optimistic leader transmits enthusiasm. Alert optimism is the best approach to life. But, the pessimist must deal with his fear.

Self awareness can make a person familiar with the fears, which rise up in his mind. This website suggests that emotions disappear, when you sense their physical symptoms. Identify the negative thoughts, which rise in your mind, when you visualize the future of your venture. Sense the symptoms of the fear, which accompany such thoughts. The emotion will be stilled. Even the fear that optimism will bring disappointment will disappear. It is a process, which takes a little practice. Freed from fear, the pessimist should focus on visualizing successful options in life. Such an approach too will soon become a "speed dial circuit" - a matter of habit.

Pessimism often follows an inability to understand the intentions and desires of other people. Some people are blessed with a mature "Theory of Mind," which understands the attitudes and behavior of people during their interactions. That creates an order in their lives by giving surrounding events purpose and meaning. When you know why something is going to happen, you can adjust better to the situation. An effective Theory of Mind is a valuable leadership skill, which grants leaders the empathic ability to imagine being in the shoes of their followers. When this skill is lacking, rude sales clerks and aggressive drivers on the road make the pessimist see a dark world. An awareness and understanding of the underlying issues of such behavior will prevent needless pessimism. Life has to be accepted as it comes, with its inevitable potholes.

"Explanatory Styles" are decided by emotions. Pessimists wince with each negative turn in life. "It is all my fault." "These things always happen to me." "Why did this have to happen to me?" "I knew this would happen to me." Such explanations of an event are triggered by persisting negative emotions. Over the longer term, such feelings can even trigger depression. If you have been a habitual pessimist, escape such torture by becoming intensely self aware. As thoughts rise, do not focus on the event, but on the nature of thoughts and feelings.

Become aware of physical symptoms of the negative feelings as and when they arise. Such awareness will still emotions over time. Stilling such emotions will transfer controls to a rational nature. Your explanatory style will change. Your mind will comfortably accept the usual setbacks in life. "What can I do now?" will then be the simple unemotional response to such events, which will prevent needless stress and illness.

Optimists emerge from setbacks with less stress than pessimists. They face problems head on and take active steps to solve problems. They are also less likely to abandon their efforts to reach their goals. But, optimism is a frame of mind, an "explanatory style," outside your conscious control. The deep intelligence within your mind has to develop new optimistic "speed dial circuits." by dwelling on the memories of your successes in life.

Dig deep into your memories and discover the times, when you succeeded, when others acknowledged your skills, or abilities. Dwell on those events. If possible, take responsibilities for the things you can do well. Deep inside, you need to become convinced of your ability to do well. Expect to discover something new and advantageous, even when you face boring, or depressing situations. A change from optimism to pessimism requires regeneration of new "speed dial circuits," which create a new explanatory style.

CHAPTER 22

# IS CONSCIOUSNESS PHYSICAL?

*"Consciousness is what makes the mind-body problem really intractable. Perhaps that is why current discussions of the problem give it little attention or get it obviously wrong."*
David Chalmers

Consciousness has long been suspected to be a spiritual or paranormal entity. Conscious awareness itself is the subjective experience of being awake and aware of one's surroundings. Its connection to the brain has confounded humanity. How can a physical organ be linked to something that is considered spiritual? This is the hard problem of consciousness. Philosophers have debated this question for centuries, with some proposing a separation between the mind and body, others denying the existence of the problem, and still others claiming that all things are conscious.

In the field of neuroscience, Francis Crick and Benjamin Libet are two names that are widely known. Crick, who is best known for his discovery of the structure of DNA along with James Watson, also made significant contributions to the study of consciousness. On the other hand, Libet was a neurophysiologist who conducted experiments on the relationship between conscious will and the brain's activity. Together, the work of Crick and Libet has greatly influenced our understanding of consciousness and the relationship between the brain and our experiences.

Francis Crick posited that the claustrum, a thin layer of gray matter in the brain, could be responsible for enabling consciousness. Consciousness allows for the integrated perception of multiple objects and events, rather than isolated attributes. The region is thought to coordinate information from various sensory domains and enable the conscious experience of perceiving integrated perceptions. When the claustrum is deactivated, the patient loses consciousness.

Conscious awareness receives observation signals from the brain, such as the decision-making process of the motor system, which can act before conscious awareness is even aware of it. Libet conducted a series of experiments in the 1980s and 1990s to study the relationship between conscious will and the brain's activity. He found that unconscious processes in the brain precede conscious decisions. The view, that conscious will is the cause of our actions, is an illusion. Libet's experiments sparked a great deal of debate and discussion in the field of neuroscience and continue to be the subject of ongoing research and investigation.

However, recent scientific findings indicate that decision making is actually a pattern recognition process in the brain. It is a purely physical phenomenon. For the Intuition Way, that intuition, which allows for rapid problem-solving, is powered by a pattern recognition algorithm. Intuition leverages vast human memories to deliver answers to complex questions in just 20 milliseconds. In reality, intuition enables the brain to identify patterns. Intuition, as a powerful pattern recognition process, enables the brain to make decisions and take actions. A similar pattern recognition process allowed AlphaGo to defeat human players in the game of Go.

Consciousness, on the other hand, merely observes these decisions and actions. It is composed mainly of intangible feelings and experiences, also known as qualia, which cannot be quantified. Millions of qualia combine to create the unique conscious experience, triggered by intuition from multiple brain regions. Qualia are triggered by the brain's pattern recognition processes in various regions, including the somesthetic association region for touch and the olfactory system for smell. The link between feelings and brain activity is well-established. The somesthetic association region of the brain uses pattern recognition to identify objects through touch.

A Nobel Prize-winning discovery established the link between the olfactory system and the sense of smell. Additionally, the motor systems in the brain make decisions and act before conscious awareness, as shown by the findings of Benjamin Libet. He discovered that motor neurons in the brain fired 350 milliseconds before a subject consciously decided to press a key. Consciousness does not act, but rather observes. Intuition, the brain's ability to quickly recognize patterns, plays a major role in conscious awareness. The brain uses this ability to make decisions and act, while conscious awareness simply observes these actions.

Many machines are designed to make decisions and take action based on pattern recognition, similar to how the brain functions. The human brain contains multiple competing intelligences, and the highest priority decision is made by one of these intelligences. Consciousness is not the decision-maker, but instead observes the decisions made by the brain. The brain makes the decisions, while conscious awareness observes and receives signals. Brain function can override conscious will, such as in the case of avoiding a risky action. Consciousness is not the decision-maker, and even one's willpower is limited by the brain's overriding priority for safety and practicality. Conscious will is merely a desire, and not the decision-maker. Intuition enables the brain to make instant decisions in just 20 milliseconds, transmitting the information to conscious awareness 350 milliseconds later. The scientific community continues to debate the spiritual nature of consciousness, but the link between the brain and consciousness is clear.

If a precise time delay can be measured between a brain action and its conscious perception, as demonstrated by Benjamin Libet, how can consciousness be considered a spiritual entity? There is scientific evidence for the physical nature of conscious awareness. The process is logically linked to pattern recognition processes and decision-making by the nervous system in the brain. In conclusion, consciousness signals are not spiritual, but instead the result of physical processes in the brain. All evidence exists to dispel the idea of conscious awareness being a spiritual or paranormal entity.

The Intuition Way is a groundbreaking work that challenges our traditional understanding of intuition. Consciousness is not a spirit, but the essence of a machine. A thermostat in a refrigerator decides when to switch on and off the compressor. Higher temperatures cause the sensing fluid to expand, and the expansion trips a switch, which shuts off electricity to the compressor. There are merely molecules responding in particular ways to the environment. A human designer structured the molecules to produce physical effects. In the case of humans, the same laws work on molecules to perceive events, record memories, recognize events, and generate physical actions to enable humans to cope with life.

The claustrum handles the feedback communication hub for the system. It is no more the seat of the soul than the thermostat. Since human communications exist in the abstract realm, people speculate that consciousness is an abstract entity, a spiritual being. However, intuition enables the prefrontal cortex to recognize that consciousness is the highest level of human intelligence. Elon Musk dreams of enabling consciousness to survive in the cosmos for future eons. Without the physical bodies, there would be no consciousness.

ABRAHAM THOMAS

www.ingramcontent.com/pod-product-compliance
Lightning Source LLC
Chambersburg PA
CBHW051559010526
44118CB00023B/2755